Make Healthcare Great Again

An *Insider's* Guide to Healthcare

Edward Shaheen, M.D.

ISBN 978-1-952827-17-4

MOM

Drake, Jax & Goblin.

CONTENTS

Acknowledgement   ix

Chapter One:
Introduction   13

Chapter Two:
The Good Ole Days of Healthcare
To Now...a Little Background   25

Chapter Three:
Insurance Companies   33

Chapter Four:
Possible Solutions to the Health
Insurance Problem   65

Chapter Five:
Employer or Direct Care Model
An Insurance Alternative   87

Chapter Six:
Physician and Non-Physician
Providers   107

Chapter Seven:
Contract Management Groups
Staffing Companies   125

Chapter Eight:
Hospitals   159

Chapter Nine:
The Pharmaceutical Industry
A.K.A. Big Pharma   189

Chapter Ten:
Government   215

Chapter Eleven:
Patients, People and the Public   263

Chapter Twelve:
Diet, Medical Marts & Simple
Package Labeling   285

Chapter Thirteen:
Technology   309

Chapter Fourteen:
Medicare for All   329

Chapter Fifteen: Conclusion   341

Glossary   349

Endnotes   359

References   367

ACKNOWLEDGEMENTS

Without question, the person in my life who emphasized the importance of health and most influenced my decision to pursue a career in medicine was my mother. She was an inspiration to me, and remains so today. Mom was a glass half-full person, tried to make the world she lived in a better place and always looked out for others. She did not expect anything in return, only hoped others would return the kindness not to her, but to others. She demonstrated unconditional love for her children and sacrificed so much so her children could have a better life. Although she has left this world, her influence continues to help others every day through her children and those who knew her. I miss you mom. Thank you, and my patients thank you.

I want to thank my four older brothers: Kay, Jim, Fred and Allen for their support and encouragement throughout my childhood, adulthood and professional life. You guys really bring meaning to what the word family should mean. No matter what, always there for each other. One sometimes can only hope to have a role model in their life, I was blessed to have five; the four of you and mom. As tough as my childhood may have been, I know it was easier than what each of you had to go through.

My oldest brother "Kay", nickname for Karim, you were like a father to the younger me. I have not forgotten that you bought me my first bike. You are the first in our family to attend college and made it much easier for the rest of the brothers to follow your example of obtaining a college degree. You were the oldest and had to go through things without an older brother to give you advice. You are incredibly tough and even when you are dealing with your medical scare and surgery, you remain brave and deal with it with great courage.

Jim, thanks for helping make my career choice so simple to make and doing all the things you could to help me be successful in my early business ventures that helped fund my college and medical school education. You have always been there for your brothers and it is much appreciated.

Fred, thank you for your support throughout my life. You helped inspire me to become something I thought I would never be, a writer. You are a great person and are one of the few people that shares the love, to the same degree, for dogs as I do.

Allen, you may be the smartest person I have ever met, period. Even though it would have been easy to tease me about it as a kid, you never did. You only encouraged me and told me I was just as smart as you. I think you must have more of a sense of humor than you get credit for. Thank you for all the help, guidance and support you have given me over the years and for taking the time to read various parts of this book and offer suggestions.

To all my teachers, professors, residency attending physicians, classmates in medical school, fellow interns and residents, senior and chief residents, off-service attending physicians, fellow physician colleagues, nurses and other health care workers who challenged, pushed, competed with, showed, encouraged, criticized, scolded and complimented me with good intentions, and sometimes not, it has been an amazing journey. By doing so, you taught me much of what I know about medicine and my specialty, pushed me to push myself to reach a higher level than I may have without you and helped mold me into a better skilled, more knowledgeable, more empathetic and more confident emergency specialist. To all of you, my brothers, and my mother, I thank you. Every patient I have seen and treated has benefitted because of you.

Lastly, and certainly not least, to all the patients I have had the pleasure and privilege of meeting, caring for and treating in my over three decades while in medical school at the University of Virginia, University Hospital, Roanoke Memorial Hospital and Blue Ridge Hospital; while completing my emergency medicine residency program at Orlando

Regional Medical Center, Sand Lake Hospital, St. Cloud Hospital and Jacksonville Memorial Medical Center; and practicing as a staff physician or medical director in Lake Charles, Louisiana; Orlando, Florida; Atlanta, Georgia; Monroe, Louisiana; Beaumont, Texas; and Ruston, Louisiana. You have taught me so much and allowed me to appreciate how fortunate I am to be trusted with something as precious and valuable as one's health. You have told me stories and I have learned lessons. We have laughed together, and we have cried together. You may have sometimes complained, but probably not as much as I might have if I were the patient. I have gained and learned so much from my patients that has allowed me to help the next patient with more wisdom, confidence and humility than my "last" patient.

Chapter One:
INTRODUCTION

Does healthcare work for you? If you are confused or angry about healthcare and the costs of healthcare, you are not alone. If you have ever received a surprise medical bill, you are not alone. If you are not sure about the safety of your local hospital, you are not alone. If you think health insurance, healthcare and understanding medical bills is complicated, you are not alone. It is confusing, complicated, and expensive. Many people who have insurance do not understand it. In fact, there are many things people do not understand about health insurance, hospitals, doctors, medications, and the many healthcare players within healthcare.

Healthcare is important to us. We need to understand it. To make good healthcare decisions, we need accurate information. Whether it is deciding what physician or hospital to choose, knowing what questions to ask doctors, hospitals, insurers or pharmacies, understanding how to obtain or negotiate lower prices; better informed consumers are better equipped to make the right decisions for themselves and their loved ones. But patients are kept in the dark and are at a disadvantage when they must make important and potentially life changing decisions.

If you want to know more about health care, so you can make wiser decisions and achieve better health, this book is for you. My name is Edward Shaheen. I have been a medical doctor for most of my life and have personally treated tens of thousands of patients during my career.

I attended the University of California at Berkeley, then a small community college, before graduating from the University of Virginia with a Bachelor Degree in Economics with Distinction. I then graduated from the University of Virginia, School of Medicine and completed my Internship and Residency at Orlando Regional Medical Center, now Orlando Health. I am a Diplomat of the American Board of Emergency Medicine and have been so since 1995. Over the past 30 years, I have been a member of numerous local, state and national medical organizations and associations at one time or another, including the American Medical Association (AMA). I have practiced medicine for over 25 years, served as Chairman of the Department of Emergency Medicine, as medical director of numerous emergency departments, on numerous hospital medical executive and other committees, task forces, foundations, and boards.

I have treated celebrities, professional athletes, famous people, but mostly people just like you and me. I have delivered babies, treated newborns, infants, children, adolescents, adults, and the elderly. I have treated patients with just about any medical condition, injury or "embarrassing situation" that you can imagine. I have treated fighter pilots, concert pianists, professional race car drivers, politicians and just about any other profession or occupation one can imagine.

I have provided expert opinion, consulting and other services to hospitals, medical groups, insurers, and Fortune 500 corporations. I have been recognized numerous times and received numerous awards. However, one of the most important credentials that I possess is that I have personally, had the trust of, and the privilege and honor to examine, treat and care for tens thousands of patients over my medical career. I have interacted with, or spoken to, hundreds of thousands of people within, related to, or associated with, medicine and healthcare over my medical career. Because of my specialty training, certifications, knowledge and experience I am recognized as an expert within my specialty.

I have witnessed a lot of things and heard a lot of stories about healthcare. I have learned a lot and accumulated much knowledge about healthcare over my career that many in the public are probably not aware. If the public was aware, people may be shocked and may make different decisions and choices when it comes to their health care i.e. how those within healthcare treat and view patients.

In this book, I will discuss health care. What is good healthcare? The many players within healthcare that have significant influence and discuss some reasons why healthcare may be the way it is i.e. broken, dysfunctional and in need of a major overhaul. I will present information from a different perspective than you may be accustomed: the perspective of the patient. A perspective that will help you better understand why things are the way they are and more importantly help you make better-informed decisions when it comes to health care and making health care decisions. From the health insurance companies, hospitals, physicians, non-physician providers, staffing companies or contract management groups (CMGs), pharmaceutical companies, retail pharmacies, medical device makers, employers, government and anyone else involved in health care with the exception of the patient or public, collectively referred to as the "Healthcare Complex," along with the public, I will discuss and explain why each player behaves the way they do. I will write why health insurance and healthcare costs so much and why care is the way it currently is. Then I will discuss some common sense and innovative ways to make healthcare great for patients and the public.

The book discusses how patients are kept in the dark about costs and the quality of the people and hospitals treating them. I will discuss the various players within the healthcare complex and introduce innovative ideas such as Lifetime Health Insurance, Health-Life Insurance policies, Direct Care Organizations (DCOs), Price-Quality Disclosures (P/Q Disclosures), Medical & Medication Menus, Policy Weakness Disclosures, D-meals, and many others.

Looking at things from a patient's perspective and, using my insight and knowledge of healthcare, the insurance industry, economics, and business, I will explain healthcare in a way that no one may have done for you before. I hope this will help you understand why things are the way they are in healthcare, so it will be easier for you to find hospitals and doctors who deliver higher quality care, find or negotiate lower prices from doctors and hospitals, pharmaceutical companies, pharmacies, insurers and others. Most importantly, the book should empower you, help you make better informed decisions and live a healthier life.

Honestly, just about anyone in healthcare stands to learn and benefit from reading this book and applying some of the common sense, innovative ideas and principals that will be discussed. The primary audience of this book is anyone who has ever been, or will ever be a patient, or anyone who is responsible for making the healthcare decisions for someone else. Having said that, each of the various players that make up the healthcare complex stand to learn and benefit from reading this book.

At times, it may seem that I am being critical of those in the healthcare complex. For those leaders, decision makers and players within the healthcare complex, you may initially not agree with me and come up with reasons that justify what you do. Deep down you may agree. I am not trying to harm you. I am trying to help you by giving you a different perspective and getting you to think in a different, more effective, efficient and patient obsessed© way. What I suggest may actually help you become more successful. If you can be introspective, and honest with yourself, you may actually realize what I discuss is true. In fact, you may realize that you, or you and the entity you represent, stand to reap great rewards by implementing some of the ideas and suggestions I present. More importantly, you can help people and be part of the solution to fixing our broken healthcare system.

If we really want to improve healthcare, we must think smart, and do things better, differently. We must be creative and innovative. We must use common sense and good judgement. No longer should we keep the patient, or the public, in the dark. We must define what is important and then focus on that. I propose defining great healthcare as keeping people healthy in both the short and the long term. To do this, we need to reset our current reward system that is built into our current healthcare system. We need to envision and create a healthcare system that align the goals, and focus, of everyone involved in healthcare on the patient and the public. We must be patient-obsessed©. Incentives and disincentives must be created and structured to reward those in healthcare when their behavior and action results in better patient and public health and outcomes and penalize those who do not act or behave in ways that improve healthcare. Our current healthcare system seems to do the opposite. In many examples, it seems to incentivize everyone in the healthcare complex to behave in a way that potentially harms healthcare and the public. We must protect the public. Those in the healthcare complex should feel a moral and ethical obligation to protect the patient and align themselves with the patients' best interest. By aligning everyone in healthcare with the same goal in mind, it will become second nature for us to behave in a manner that should result in much better results, i.e. better outcomes, less days of illness, less days lost from work, etc. and much lower costs. Incentives and disincentives must apply to everyone involved in healthcare to encourage better choices. I will offer some examples of possible incentives and disincentives in this book that may help accomplish this goal for those within healthcare.

I challenge the public, the biggest user of healthcare, and those who may influence healthcare: patients, family members, employers, insurers, hospitals, physicians and other non-physician healthcare providers, lawmakers, etc. to make healthcare great again. While this book is not intended to have all the answers to our healthcare dilemma, or the exact roadmap to fixing everything, it presents information and ideas that can make a difference, help fix our broken healthcare system and improve the quality of life of our citizens. Some of these ideas are innovative and the result of much thought after applying common sense to the knowledge and experience I have accumulated over my career. I will discuss ideas to think about, changes we can make to improve treatments and care, save money, and most importantly help make us be healthier so we can avoid or minimize suffering, illness, and pain. Let us shed light on the darkness the healthcare complex casts on the public and empower you with information and knowledge that will allow you to make better informed decisions for you and your family.

In the coming pages and chapters, I will discuss the various players within healthcare. I will try to explain who the various players are, what they do and why they behave in the manner they do. The book will look at some possible ways to improve these players' behavior and align them with what is best for patients. The hope is that you will learn important and useful information about our current healthcare system and allow you to understand healthcare from a new or different perspective.

This book may make you aware of things you are completely unaware of or help reinforce things that you may already know or wonder about regarding healthcare. It will provide you with some information, thoughts, knowledge, concepts, and ideas that might help you view things differently. Hopefully, it will inspire and empower you. Hopefully, it will influence all the players within the healthcare system to change their actions and behavior in order to fix our current broken healthcare system and ultimately help us make healthcare great again for patients and all of us.

I will discuss information that will help address such questions such as:

- What is healthcare?
- Why is our healthcare system the way it is?
- Why our current system is not better?
- Why the various people and entities within healthcare (the "players") do what they do?
- What are some creative, different, or innovative ways to align those within healthcare with what is best for the patient?
- How to design a system that will inspire those within healthcare to behave in a manner that can help the patient, the insured, the public and society.

I will present some ideas that could make healthcare better. Creative and innovative concepts and ideas will be introduced and discussed. The hope is you will learn useful and valuable information that will help you make better informed decisions that will help make our current broken healthcare system better and ultimately help you, your family and society as a whole live healthier lives.

Depending on your role in healthcare, this book could help you if you are:

- A patient or decision maker for a patient who wants to live a healthier life, be better able to afford healthcare or save money on your healthcare.
- A parent concerned about a child
- A mother who makes health decisions for the whole family
- A child concerned about a parent
- A physician or non-physician provider, it could help improve communication to patients and improve patient compliance, help grow your practice or increase revenue and profits.
- A hospital CEO, or administrator who wants to improve the services offered to the community you serve or improve the fiscal health of your hospital or health care organization.
- An insurance executive who wants to really help the insured and wants to maximize your company's long term profits
- An owner, or leader, of a staffing company or contract management group (CMG) who wants to improve the value the staffing company delivers to patients and client hospitals, improve physician retention and morale or increase long term revenues or profits for the CMG.
- A pharmaceutical executive who genuinely wants to help people and do good for humanity
- An employer looking for ways to help your employees, lessen the number of sick days, improve morale for your employees, lower healthcare costs and improve your "bottom line"
- A person who likes to learn, understand or be able to help others
- A government leader interested in better serving your constituents and looking for ways to do it

- Any other player in the healthcare complex who wants to do good, lower the costs of care or improve the health of patients and the public

If any of the above happen to describe you, this book is for you. The information, examples, concepts and ideas I will discuss may give you a better understanding of healthcare from a perspective you may not have considered. This book may help you accomplish what may be important to you. The difference is this book provides some guidance on how to accomplish many of these things by doing what is best for the patient, not at the expense of the patient.

In *Make Healthcare Great Again*, I will discuss some commonly used terms and some new, creative terms and ideas. For your convenience, at the end of each chapter I list some of the important ideas or "Talking Points" discussed in that chapter. Also, I have included a glossary at the end of the book that serves as a reference, to help make it easier to understand the meaning of certain terms.

In this book, to some there may be times when what is written may come off as politically incorrect, harsh, inconsiderate, or offensive. It is not my intention to offend anyone, be offensive or cruel. I am not a mean, uncompassionate person. To the contrary, I want what is best and fair for patients, people, and society. I tend to be a straight-forward, no-nonsense person when it comes to solving problems. While emotions are natural and can be good, they often can cloud judgment and lead us to decisions we later regret. Political correctness can also prevent us from making the most effective decisions and changes that we must make. One must understand and accept that disease, illness, and facts are not emotional or politically correct. Things, sometimes, are what they are. One must understand that sometimes bad things happen to humans regardless of our age, sex, race, country of national origin, sexual orientation, political affiliation, economic status, state of fitness, height, weight, eye color, hair color or any other similar or unique quality we as individuals possess.

Illness, disease injury and suffering are the enemy. People get sick and injured, suffer, and die. Unfortunately, human nature often requires bad things to occur to us before human behavior will change. When people finally start changing as a result of the bad things that have happened to us, society benefits. Perhaps that is because we do not make the right decisions ahead of time, before bad things happen, because doing so is undesirable, may be unpopular or perceived as politically incorrect. Humans are flawed in this way. We often cannot do the right thing i.e. quit smoking, eat healthier, manage our chronic illnesses, suggest to a loved one or patient to lose weight, etc. to prevent bad from happening. People sometimes must wait for bad things to happen to them before they finally act and change. Even then, some people still do not change their behavior.

Even when we do things intended to help, to prevent suffering or avoid hurting someone's feelings, we sometimes end up doing harm to the ones we intended to help. So, if there is something offensive that could have been stated more politically correct, or seems harsh, it is not intentional. My intentions are to help educate, clearly make a point or to help you better understand the subject matter. It is hoped and believed that you, regardless of who you are, will learn and benefit from reading this book and feel challenged, inspired and empowered to help make healthcare better for yourself, your family, your practice, your company, your constituency, your hospital or organization, and by doing so, for all of us. By doing so we can fix our current broken healthcare system, help ourselves, help patients, help society, and empower you to make better informed healthcare decisions and live a healthier life.

I hope you enjoy reading this book and learn information that will improve your health. Hopefully, it will help you help me impact and help more people than I would ever be able to do alone. Regardless of who you are, I hope you find my observations, experiences, reporting and opinion insightful and helpful. Not everyone may agree with everything in this book and that is OK. So long as it stimulates thought and inspires you to be better informed or do something that will improve your health or the health of others, the time spent writing this book was worth the effort. If you like this book, find the information in it to be useful, interesting, valuable, enlightening or it helps you or yours live a healthier life, save money or helps in any other way, I ask that you spread the word and tell others about it. The more people who become informed and empowered, the better off we are as individuals and as a nation. I would love to hear from you, so please let me know what you think of my book. Any, and all, comments are welcomed. E-mail me at 2020MHGA@gmail.com. Thank you, and I wish you great health.

After you finish this book, if you are a current or future patient, a family member of a patient or a decision maker for anyone, it is my hope that you will:

- No longer be kept in the dark by the healthcare complex about anything to do with your healthcare.
- Be better informed and understand the current healthcare system and why it is how it is.
- Know what to expect when interacting with any player in the healthcare complex and have informative, useful and meaningful conversations with them.
- Understand what is reasonable to demand from the healthcare system and the players within it.
- Know what questions to ask of doctors, hospital representative, insurers, etc.
- Know what to look for and how to obtain better care.
- Be able to have meaningful conversations with friends, family, co-workers, employers, employees, neighbors, patients, or anyone else.
- Understand how to look for lower prices or negotiate better rates with hospitals, physicians, pharmaceutical companies and others.
- Understand how to help change healthcare for the better.
- Learn information and have talking points so you are able to spread useful and accurate information to others to help them

make better informed healthcare related decisions, and most of all,

- Be empowered to make better decisions and choices in healthcare and to live healthier, happier lives.

Edward Shaheen, M.D.

Chapter Two:

THE GOOD OLE DAYS OF HEALTHCARE...A LITTLE BACKGROUND

Once upon a time, health insurance was great; any illness or injury was covered. People felt safe and secure that they could get the testing, care, and treatment they need should they become sick or injured. Once upon a time, health insurance was affordable. Policies were provided by employers or bought directly by the public at a low price. Policies had a low deductible, or no deductible at all. People believed that should they get sick or injured, they would only have to worry about getting better. The health insurance policy meant something and would be welcomed by just about any doctor or hospital. They trusted that not only their doctor but also their health insurer, hospital, and everyone else involved in healthcare were most concerned with their health and well-being. Health insurance was simple. There was little or no confusion or issues about in-network or out-of-network, co-pays, co-insurance, waiting periods or pre-existing conditions. People seemed to be in better health then. People ate healthier and many lived healthier lifestyles. Less people got sick and when they did, they received quality care and great service. People knew if they had "good health insurance," they would not have to worry so much about paying for healthcare costs should they get sick or injured. Medical bills did not commonly create financial stress or cause families to file for bankruptcy.

In the past decade, things have changed considerably. Healthcare costs have skyrocketed, outpacing wages and inflation rates by almost 100%.[1] Employer based health insurance policy rates had double-digit annual increases during the 2000-2010 period.[2] Less people have employer sponsored health insurance and more of the costs have been shifted to the employee. Low or zero-dollar deductible plans are disappearing, not available or are cost prohibited. According to the Kaiser Family Foundation Employer Health Benefits Survey, in 2018, 85% of employee insurance plans have deductibles. This is about a 50% increase just in the last 10 years.[3] Deductibles of employer-based insurance are 212% of what they were 10 years ago.[4] Health plans are more complicated, confusing and most people do not fully understand their coverage. People are not well-informed about healthcare and seem to make poor choices when it comes to maintaining good health. Costs have gotten so out of control that healthcare costs often wipe out a family's savings or lead patients to declare bankruptcy. If healthcare costs continue to increase as they have, it could lead to crisis that could match or exceed the financial meltdown that occurred with the housing meltdown of the late 2000's. Medicare A is at risk of having to cut benefits by 10-15% by 2028[5]. According to the Committee for Responsible Federal Budget's (CRFB) May 16, 2018 report:

> "In 2017, the United States spent about $3.5 trillion, or 18% of its gross domestic product (GDP), on health expenditures-more than twice the average of developed countries. Of that, $3.5 trillion, $1.5 trillion is directly or indirectly financed by the federal government. In other words, the federal government dedicates resources of nearly 8 percent of the economy toward health care."[6]

The CRFB adds that "rising healthcare costs represent a threat to both the Medicare program and the federal budget more broadly."[7] If things do not change, our nation's debt will become unsustainable and our economic stability could be threatened or destroyed.

Population health is important and is receiving more and more attention in government and the media. Healthy people are more productive and contribute to the betterment of society. Healthy people are more likely to be employed and produce goods and services that are desired and benefit society. Aside from that, healthcare is big business.

This is part of the reason that healthcare has been a topic of conversation. Healthcare costs make up a large percentage of our country's GDP (gross domestic product). Using an estimated population of 329,345,233,[8] over $10,000/person per year, on average, is spent on healthcare for each man, woman and child in America. About one in every six dollars spent in the United States is healthcare related. For employer funded employee healthcare family plans, it is estimated that about $20,000 per employee is spent on healthcare, when one includes employee family policy premiums, co-pays, co-insurance, deductibles, prescriptions and other costs.[9] On an individual level, healthcare costs are often responsible for financial hardship and bankruptcy in our country.

The United States has the best medical treatment in the world but not the best healthcare

We hear stories about how people from many other countries travel to the US for surgery or treatment. Mick Jagger, the lead singer for the Rolling Stones band, someone with the enough money and resources to have treatment anywhere in the world, recently came to the US to have successful heart surgery. World leaders come to the United States to receive care and treatment for a variety of ailments. Ask people, who has the best healthcare in the world, and many will say the United States. I respectfully disagree. According to a Commonwealth Fund publication comparing 11 industrialized countries, the United States ranked dead last behind England, Germany, the Netherlands, New Zealand, Australia, Canada, France, Norway, Sweden and Switzerland.[10] One could make the argument that our healthcare system is a disaster, even a failure in many regards. The United States spends about 17.8% of its gross domestic product (GDP) on healthcare while the other 10 nations listed and ranked ahead of the US only spent on average 11.5% of their GDP on healthcare.[11]

Our healthcare system is broken. It is getting worse, more complicated and expensive. The United States has the best medical treatment in the world but not the best healthcare. To some this may sound like the same thing, but it is not.

Healthcare is complex but it does not have to be complicated. In fact, it should be simple. The simpler the better. This is an important concept to remember. The simpler something is, the easier it will be to understand, and the more likely more people will be able to understand and benefit. If incentives and disincentives for everyone involved in healthcare are designed to maximize great health for people now and in the long term, these incentives and disincentives would influence behaviors for the better, and we could immediately see changes that would actually result in a great healthcare system that benefits everyone, including and most importantly, the patient and the public in general.

I will use the term **"Healthcare Complex."** The healthcare complex includes everyone within the healthcare system except the patients and their families. It is intended to include insurance companies, hospitals, pharmaceutical companies, pharmacy benefit managers, retail pharmacies, medical device makers, physicians, non-physician providers such as nurse practitioners and physician assistants, imaging centers, laboratories, government, and just about any other company, person or entity involved in healthcare except the patient.

When I use the term **"Healthcare System,"** I am referring to everyone in the healthcare complex plus the patient, their families and the public. We currently have a healthcare system where the public and the patients are sitting ducks and at the mercy of the healthcare complex. The public is set up to be taken advantage of by the healthcare complex "players." For those of you who play or understand poker, let me use this analogy. It's as if the patient is playing poker with the various players in the healthcare complex but all the healthcare complex players can see the patient's cards but the patient cannot see the other players' card nor does the patient understand the cards he has or the rules of the game. These healthcare players keep the patient and public in the dark regarding quality, pricing and many options that may be available. Members of this healthcare complex make fortunes while the patient pays more and gets less.

Healthcare is complex but it does not have to be complicated

Our healthcare system is broken and has been for some time. Perhaps a better name for our current healthcare system is "sick care" rather than healthcare. Most of our "health" care comes into play after we get sick. The healthcare complex financially benefits when people get sick and need care or treatment, not when they are "healthy." In our current broken healthcare system, prevention is not rewarded enough. If the public stays healthy, many in the healthcare complex would lose money or may go out of business. Except for insurance companies, the financial incentive to the healthcare complex players occurs only after a person becomes ill or injured. From the healthcare complex players' perspective, there is little to no financial incentive to prevent people from ever getting ill or injured. Most of their income comes from treating people who are sick or injured, not preventing illness or promoting good health. Historically, the big money has been in treatment i.e. cardiac bypass surgery, cancer treatment, joint replacements, spine or neurosurgery, medical devices, prescription drugs, etc. Think about it. Think of all the advertising you see regarding cancer treatment or cancer centers, cardiac and orthopedic surgery, various medications to treat diseases and various illnesses. Why are these services and products promoted so heavily by hospitals and pharmaceutical companies? Why are cardiac surgeons and cardiologists paid so much more than other physicians? They generate lots of money for the hospitals that have cardiac surgery and cardiology services. Why do you think oncologists make so much money? Orthopedic surgeons? Neurosurgeons? You get the idea. Primary care physicians (PCPs) on the other hand, typically make only a fraction of what these specialists make yet they have great potential to positively impact healthcare and prevent illness from ever occurring. They may be able to help prevent more illness and suffering than the many specialists who get paid 2, 3 even 10 times more.

When I think of great healthcare, I imagine a system that enables people to avoid, or minimize, illness and sickness.

Based on income of PCPs, it does not appear that prevention of all the pain and suffering (and financial costs) associated with diseases and other illnesses is valued the same as treating those patients who become ill or sick. So, does society really value healthcare as much as we think? Based on this example of income disparities, one could argue that society seems to place value on helping the sick getting better, not keeping healthy people from becoming sick. What ever happened to the saying "an ounce of prevention is worth a pound of cure?"

Healthcare must be more than patient-focused, it needs to be patient-obsessed©

What is goal of healthcare? Is it better to be able to treat someone when they get sick or is it better to avoid ever getting sick in the first place and never needing treatment? When I think of great healthcare, I imagine a system that enables people to avoid, or minimize, illness and sickness. A system in which:

- Anyone who is sick or injured can obtain the best available treatment to get well again quickly, easily, and effectively.
- Access to quality healthcare would be easy with minimal obstacles and fast to obtain
- People would have their choice as to what doctor or non-physician provider they want to see, what hospital or facility at which they want to be treated and how they are treated.

- The cost to see whatever physician or non-physician provider they want is fair and known ahead of time and to all.
- Healthcare must be more than patient-focused, it needs to be **patient-obsessed©**. Whatever is best for the patient in terms of quality, convenience, service, price and outcomes would be the highest priority. This applies on both an individual health and population health level.

In a sense, when someone gets sick, the healthcare system has already failed. The system then provides treatment to try and mitigate the damage that has incurred. Instead of waiting for the population to become sick and then measuring how effective treatment is, we should measure:

- How infrequently people do get sick?
- The overall number of healthy days or years not requiring unexpected treatment? I.e. number of days without lost day of work.
- How many people are healthy and the factors responsible for keeping them healthy?

This is not to say we should not track and grade the effectiveness of treatment when someone becomes ill. Of course, there may be other factors affecting one's health, but perhaps we can improve our healthcare significantly and certainly should be able to lower the cost without worsening the outcomes. In fact, we should be able to improve the health of our population and save billions, even trillions of dollars, as we do it.

Chapter 2 Talking Points:

- Healthcare is important because keeping people healthy can save a lot of human suffering and a lot of money.
- The United States spends $3.5 Trillion on healthcare. If costs continue to rise at their current pace, healthcare costs could lead to the financial collapse of Medicare and threaten America's economic stability.
- Great Healthcare places an emphasis on the prevention of illness, but should someone become ill, would provide:
    - Patient choice of doctor, hospital or other facility and treatment
    - Easy access to quality care
    - Fair, transparent and affordable costs

Chapter Three:

INSURANCE COMPANIES

A Little History-Background

The concept behind insurance is to spread risk to allow people to have some sense of safety or security. Let's use a simple example of fire insurance. Homes burn down on occasion, but it is very unlikely that any one person's home will burn down in any given year. Yet, if a person happens to be the unfortunate one who's home burns down, that person would likely be financially devastated. So, for society to spread out risk and protect whoever may lose their home to fire, everyone "chips" into a fund to help rebuild homes that burn down i.e. fire insurance. If 1 out of 10,000 homes burn down each year and the average home costs $300,000 to rebuild, and if every one of those 10,000 homeowners pay $50 a year into this fund for the security of knowing their house will be rebuilt should it burn down, there will be $500,000 available each year to build a new home per every 10,000 homeowners; enough to cover the cost of rebuilding the home that burned down. This "chipping in" is how the risk of the single homeowner who has their home burn down is spread out to everyone who "chipped in" $50 to protect them for a potential $300,000 loss or expense. That is the concept of insurance and how it spreads the risk out. The more likely a "hazard" or bad occurrence occurs, the more expensive the chipping in amount i.e. insurance premium, is likely to be.

Health insurance is no different. If one knows they are going to be healthy and not need any care or treatment, then it would be financially unwise to have insurance. There would be no reason to pay for something that one does not need or use.

In a sense, when someone gets sick, the healthcare system has already failed

Because healthcare can be very expensive and we cannot be sure we will not require treatment or care i.e. things sometimes happen unexpectedly, we pay for insurance with the understanding that should something happen i.e. we get sick or injured, we will have insurance that will cover the expenses of any needed treatment and not cause financial ruins. Even though health insurance can seem very expensive, it can be much less than the costs of healthcare for certain conditions or illnesses. The treatment costs of certain cancers, surgeries, transplants and treatments can easily run into the hundreds of thousands of dollars. Few people can afford such massive costs.   Fortunately for most people, large catastrophic or serious health issues are relatively uncommon. Insurance companies base their business model on risk and the costs, should a hazard occur. So long as insurance companies can:

- Predict the likelihood of something happening
- Predict he likely cost should it occur
- Charge enough to cover these predicable costs, costs associated with administering their service and a little extra for a safe margin of error and profit

Insurance companies should make a handsome profit. This is how they make money. Insurers use what are called actuarial tables and formulas that predicts the likelihood of someone requiring health care and that helps them predict how expensive an individual will be to cover. Factor's that insurers use to calculate the risk of insuring a person include but are not limited to:

- Age
- Gender
- Tobacco use or abstinence
- Medical history
- Family history

- Occupation

These factors help the insurance underwriters, people who determine risks based on actuarial tables and information specific to a person, calculate the likelihood of a person using healthcare services and thus helps predict how much it will cost the insurer to cover an individual. Once calculated, the insurer will determine whether to offer insurance or not and how much to charge someone should they be offered coverage.

The average annual premium for health insurance in 2018 was $6,896 for single coverage and $19,616 for family coverage[12]

Typically, the insurer will offer coverage for a term of one year at a set price. It is quite common for this price to go up every year. In some cases, insurance companies will determine someone is too expensive, or high risk, to be insured and will not offer insurance coverage to them. If someone uses up lots of healthcare because of a new diagnosis or unfortunate illness or accident, providing coverage to that person is more likely to cause the insurance company to lose money on the coverage. If someone already has health issues, known as a "pre-existing condition," and will require more care than another person, the individual with a pre-existing conditions is expected to cost more to the insurer than that same person if they did not have a pre-existing condition. In such cases, the insurer may determine that the person is too high a risk and decide not to renew their coverage (drop them) after the current term is up. So long as insurers take in more in health insurance premiums then they must pay out for care and all other expenses, they are profitable. The insurance industry's practice of dropping or not insuring people with pre-existing conditions was addressed by the Affordable Care Act (ACA), "Obama Care." The ACA no longer allowed insurers to deny health insurance coverage to someone because they had a pre-existing health condition. This and allowing children to remain on their parents' health insurance until age 26 are two of the most popular things about the ACA.

The average dollar amount contributed by the employee was $1,186 for single coverage and $5,547 for family coverage[13]

Other than spreading risk amongst their many policy holders, another intended advantage of the existence of health insurers is for them to serve as a "watchdog" of many within the healthcare complex and patients. The idea is insurers will negotiate lower prices with hospitals, doctors, pharmaceutical companies and others in the healthcare complex in order to keep healthcare costs down for consumers, employers and the public. The insurers will also determine whether the care the insured person is seeking is warranted. If not, the insurance company will not pay for the care or service the patient is seeking or has already received i.e. deny authorization or payment. While a great concept, it seems the insurance industry has failed to produce good results. According to the 2018 Kaiser Family Foundation (KFF) Employer Health Survey:

> "The average annual premium in 2018 of private employer-sponsored health insurance plans, which covers approximately 152 million people, was $6,896 for single coverage and $19,616 for family coverage. On average, the employee contributed 18% of the premium for single coverage plans and 29% for family coverage plans. Annually, the average dollar amount contributed by the employee was $1,186 for single coverage and $5,547 for family coverage. This is an increase of 65% since 2008 and 21% since 2013, far exceeding the increases in wages during the same period. This seems to be a reoccurring problem. From 2000-2006, employer sponsored health insurance family coverage premiums increased by 78%, while wages only increased 20%; between 2006 and 2012, premiums

increased by 37%, while wages increased by 18%; and between 2012 and 2018, premiums increased by 25%, while wages increased by 14%. While the good news is that the difference seems to be narrowing, the bad news is that insurance premiums are still increasing over 75% faster than wages. In addition to premiums, there are additional costs to workers for deductibles, co-pays and co-insurance. Average deductibles in employer sponsored insurance plans for all workers have increased over 53% in the past five (5) years. Over 60% of workers must pay a copayment when they see a primary care physician or specialist and about 25% of all workers must pay coinsurance (a percentage of covered amount) when the covered worker sees a primary care doctor (24%) or specialist (27%)."[14]

Unless insurance companies are very bad at predicting costs on a consistent basis, they usually make a lot of money. If one pays attention to the various articles in print and online, one might see: "Health Insurer Anthem's Profit, 2018 Forecast Top Estimates;"[15] "Blue Cross Posts 2nd-Highest Profit in Past Decade (March 1, 2019);"[16] "Cigna Boosts 2018 Forecast After Third Quarter Earnings Beat (November 1, 2018);"[17] and "Humana Profits Top Estimates...."[18] "Cigna Reported a Near 38 Percent Net Rise in Income For Shareholders..."[19]

Have you ever been to a big city with tall buildings on the skyline and paid attention to the names that are on these buildings? There are a lot of insurance company names on them: BC/BS (Blue Cross/Blue Shield), Aetna, United Healthcare, the list goes on. As you can see in Table 1, Health insurance is big business. According to Forbes, the 2018 revenue for the top eight (8) health insurers by membership were as follows:[20]

Table 1:

Insurer	Revenue in 2018
United	$201,000,000,000.00

Health	
Anthem	$ 90,000,000,000.00
Aetna	$ 60,600,000,000.00
Cigna	$ 41,600,000,000.00
Humana	$ 53,700,000,000.00
Centene	$ 48,300,000,000.00
Molina Healthcare	$ 18,800,000,000.00
WellCare Health Plans	$ 16,900,000,000.00

According to Forbes list of top 20 companies in 2018 Revenue, UnitedHealth ranks sixth (6th) in revenue, only behind Walmart-$514B, Exxon Mobil-$290B, Apple $265, Berkshire Hathaway-$247B and Amazon-$232.[21] These companies typically have CEOs that answer to stockholders who want to make money. It seems insurers are more interested in making money than doing the "right thing." This is part of the problem. And by the "right thing," I am referring to doing what is in the best interest of the policy holder or patient. Another simple way of defining the right thing is what someone's mother might say is the right thing to do? Insurers often deny payment for care that treating physicians believe are necessary even though insurers are not trained or qualified as physicians and do not examine or treat the patients.

About 60% of Americans struggle to cover a $500 emergency expense and the CEO of a single health insurance company makes 43,000 times more than that in a single year

The executives of insurance companies make obscene amounts of money compared to "regular" hard-working people. The combined compensation for just five (5) executives of United Health for fiscal year 2018 was over $68 million.[22] The median employee pay at UnitedHealth was $57,412 in 2018; David Wichmann's 2018 total compensation, the CEO of United Health, was $21.5 million or 316 times more than the median employee's income.[23] In 2014, Stephen J. Hemsley, who was CEO of UnitedHealth Group at that time, received $66.13 million in compensation.[24] Forbes reports that "63% of Americans Don't Have Enough Savings to cover a $500 Emergency."[25] A Money magazine article indicates that "40% of Americans Can't cover a $400 Emergency Expense."[26] CNBC published an article indicating "Millions of Americans Are Only $400 Away From Financial Hardship."[27] About 60% of Americans struggle to cover a $500 emergency expense and the CEO of a single health insurance company makes 43,000 times more than that in a single year. One can understand the public's outrage and why many believe health insurance companies, and those who run them, are greedy and out of touch.

One would think that with insurance companies making so much money, insurers would lower premiums, or pay for the healthcare costs, of their insured. Well, this is not the case. Insurance companies often deny payments of the healthcare expenses incurred by the insured. Is this because the medical treatment is not necessary or reasonable, or could it be to increase profits of the insurer? Other times, insurers require the patient to pay a percentage of the costs (co-insurance). Other times even if the care or treatment is covered, they will require the patient to pay the first five, ten or twenty thousand dollars (deductible) before the insurer pays a dime. Insurers get more and more creative to find reasons not to pay for, or pay a lower percentage of, the healthcare expenses of the people that trusted them to pay for these very expenses in the first place.

Insurers seem more interested in making profits and are driven to look for ways to increase/maximize profits. So, when an insurer denies making a payment for an expense incurred by a patient, that money can go towards profits. This seems to be the opposite of doing what is best for people and patients. Doctors are supposed to look out for the best interests of patients; doctors take an oath to do no harm. No one said insurers are supposed to look after the best interests of customers/insured. I am not aware of a Hippocratic Oath of insurers to protect the insured as a priority. So, when there is a discrepancy about whether a certain test, treatment or procedure is necessary, where the attending physician states it is needed and the insurer states it is not, who should we trust? Who would you want to decide? Your doctor who is seeing, examining and treating you, who has taken an oath to do no harm and tries to help patients, or your insurer who tries to maximize profits in order to please its shareholders?

Insurance companies sell their insurance policies to the public. These policies are quite long, contain many terms foreign to many in the public and are rather confusing to even the most educated. Keep in mind, many of us that comprise the public, and are customers of insurers, are not sophisticated enough to fully understand the contents of the insurance policies. Whether due to poor judgment, embarrassment, lack of time, misplaced trust or other reasons, the public buys insurance policies that it does not understand. People do not know what would happen, what would be covered, what would be denied and what the costs to the patient would be should the need for care or treatment arise.

Some might argue that the public does indeed understand insurance and what they are buying very well. I respectfully disagree. If someone truly understands something, they should be able to explain it to others and answer most any questions that one might have about it. So, I challenge the insurers to demonstrate that their customers can explain the policies that they have. Are the insured able to not only say how much the policy costs, which is often the biggest reason for selecting a policy over another, but also explain what the deductible, co-pay and co-insurance is on that policy and what does it mean? In plain English, how much will you have to pay?

- If you must go to the ER for a car accident?
- If your child is running a fever and vomiting in the middle of the night and you seek medical attention?
- If you have the worst headache of your life and go to the ER?

If the total ER bill is $12,000:

- How much will you be responsible to pay?
- Will you get a "surprise" bill?
- Will the policyholder be able to give accurate answers to these questions?

If not, then the policyholder does not fully understand the policy and the insurer has failed you, the other healthcare players and the public. Will you know?

- Whether the hospital, ER doctor, the radiologist who reads the images, the anesthesiologist that may be involved or other physician and non-physician providers are in, or out of, network?
- What contracts the insurer has or does not have with the various physician and non-physician providers?
- That the insurer may refuse to pay for tests, procedures and care that the insurance company determines were not needed or authorized?
- You might have to pay for these out-of-pocket?
- How much of what you pay will count towards your deductible?
- Whether the insurer is likely not to pay a single penny until the full amount of the deductible is paid by the policyholder?

Deductibles can be in the thousands, or tens of thousands, of dollars. According to information presented at the American College of Emergency Physician's Leadership Advocacy Conference held in Washington D.C in May 2019, a typical private insurance deductible is $7,000. Out of curiosity, you may want to check your insurance card. Is the deductible amount printed on your insurance card? Some insurers print it on insurance cards, some don't. Ever wonder why? Is your total out of pocket costs listed?

Insurers sell insurance plans that cost a lot of money. One can argue that some policies are worse than no insurance at all. Let me give an example. Most people have limited resources and must make choices on how to spend the limited money or resources they have. People choose to buy health insurance so they can get the care they need and avoid having to pay high medical expenses associated with medical treatment that could cause significant financial stress or lead to bankruptcy. The problem is a patient with a high deductible plan may not be able to afford to use the insurance that he spent thousands on. Unless he has additional money to cover the deductible, he may not receive treatment and the insurance company won't pay a dime. An uninsured patient who has not spent thousands on insurance premiums at least may have what he saved in insurance premium payments to use to pay for his healthcare.

Insurance companies offer all sorts of plans at many prices. Unfortunately, since many people do not understand exactly what they are buying, they often choose plans based on cost and not coverage. They may know it is insurance, but they do not understand or know the specifics of the following:

1) How much is the policy limit is?
2) How much is the annual policy limit?
3) How much is the lifetime limit?
4) What does in-network and out-of-network mean?
5) Is my doctor in network?
6) What doctors are in-network?
7) What hospitals are in-network?
8) If a hospital is in-network, does that mean all physicians at that hospital are also in-network?
9) Will my current doctor accept this insurance?
10) What is a pre-existing condition?
11) Does my insurance cover my condition?
12) Is my condition considered pre-existing?

13) How much is the deductible for a hospital visit for an in-network hospital?
14) How much is the deductible for a hospital visit for an out of network hospital?
15) How much is the deductible for an in-network ER visit?
16) How much is the deductible for an out of network ER visit?
17) How much is the deductible for an in-network primary care visit?
18) How much is the deductible for an out of network primary care visit?
19) How much is the deductible for an in-network urgent care visit?
20) How much is the deductible for an out of network urgent care visit?
21) How much is the co-pay for an in-network ER visit?
22) How much is the co-pay for an out of network ER visit?
23) How much is the co-pay for an in-network primary care visit?
24) How much is the co-pay for an out of network primary care visit?
25) How much is the co-pay for an in-network urgent care visit?
26) How much is the co-pay for an out of network urgent care visit?
27) How much is co-insurance for an in-network ER visit?
28) How much is the co-insurance for an out of network ER visit?
29) How much is the co-insurance for an in-network primary care visit?
30) How much is the co-insurance for an out of network primary acre visit?
31) How much is the co-insurance for an in-network primary care visit?
32) How much is the co-insurance for an out of network primary care visit?
33) Does my insurance cover prescription medications?
34) How much is the co-pay for prescription medications?
35) Is there a co-insurance for prescription medications?
36) How much is the deductible for medications?
37) How much does policy limit mean?
38) What is a deductible?
39) What is co-insurance?
40) What is a co-pay?
41) How much will I have to pay if I go to the doctor?
42) How much will I have to pay if someone in my family gets sick?
43) How much will I have to pay if I need expensive surgery?
44) What is the total amount I will have to pay in any given year?
45) Am I able to negotiate my co-pay, co-insurance or deductible with the doctor or hospital?
46) How much will I have to pay for a $12,000 ER visit?
47) How much will I have to pay for a $50,000 observation or overnight stay?

48) How much will I have to pay for a $100,000 surgery?
49) How much will I have to pay for a $1,000,000 prolonged hospitalization and treatment?

These are just some of the many things that can be confusing. There are many other questions I could list. While this list might be overkill, I could have listed many more. I intentionally listed and numbered as many as I did to give you a visual illustration of exactly how ridiculous things are and how confusing insurance companies make understanding health insurance. It's absurd for insurance companies to believe that insurance policies are simple to understand and that everyone understands exactly what is covered and not covered in any situation.

If you have a health insurance policy and don't fully understand it, you are not alone. I wish I could give you the specific answer to each of the questions I just listed. The answer to these questions is: it depends. It depends on the specific terms of the insurance policy that you have. There are many different policies from many health insurers that have different terms and clauses regarding what is covered. Depending on the policy, the amounts for the various costs that the policy holder is responsible can vary. In fact, the same insurer has many different policies with different amounts for deductibles, co-pays, etc. While I cannot explain exactly what your insurance amounts and limits are without seeing the specific policy, I can try to explain what some of the many common insurance terms used mean. Some of the more common terms used by insurance companies include but are not limited to:

- Premiums
- Deductibles
- Co-pays
- Co-insurance
- In-network or out-of-network
- Maximum out of pocket
- Policy limit
- Pre-existing conditions and
- Eligible services or charges

The following is not intended to be a comprehensive discussion or cover every aspect of each term but instead a general overview as many insurance policies are different and have different terms, requirements, exceptions and language. This is part of the reason why insurance policies are so hard to explain without reading the particulars of the actual policy. The terms, language and exceptions can be very complicated and confusing. The following explanation may be an over-simplification but is intended to help with the understanding of the terms. Hopefully, it will give a general idea of the terms. Any examples used are hypothetical and are used only to try to convey a point. Keep in mind, I am not aware that any of these policy holder obligations i.e. deductibles, co-pays, etc. are required under law. It is my understanding that these terms were invented by the insurance company and their inclusion in health insurance policies shift more of the financial responsibility of healthcare expenses away from insurers and back onto the public. It also serves as a great way for insurance company to increase their profits. If you have any questions or want a specific answer, contact your insurance company, a healthcare attorney, or a trusted professional healthcare expert.

A **premium** is the cost of the insurance policy. This is the amount that the consumer pays or that is paid on behalf of the consumer. Often, employers will pay all, or a significant part, of the insurance premium for an employee to be covered by the health insurance plan. For simplicity and the purposes of this discussion, we will say the patient or consumer pays the premium even though employers contribute. This is the minimum amount that the consumer will pay each year for healthcare. Even if the insured does not require any treatment, medication or ever sees a doctor, the premium is paid. Any other required payments by the patient are in addition to the premium. i.e. deductibles, co-pays, co-insurance and non-eligible or non-covered services charges.

A **deductible** is the amount, in addition to the insurance premiums, that the patient must pay before the insurance company will be responsible for any part of the healthcare costs by an insured customer. With few exceptions, the policyholder will always have to pay the full deductible before the insurance company will pay any amount. Customer and patient are used interchangeably. Deductible amounts vary. The higher the deductible, the more the patient will have to pay out of pocket before the insurance company will pay any amount. All other things being equal, the higher the deductible, the more likely the insurance premium will be lower. The lower the deductible, the higher the insurance premium is likely to be. Insurance companies sell policies with deductibles as low as $0, no deductibles, or as high as in the thousands or tens of thousands of dollars or more. If a customer has a policy with a $5,000 deductible and receives medical care that costs $4,000, the patient will likely have to pay the entire $4,000 out of pocket. The insurance company will pay nothing. The insurance company is not required to pay anything until the full amount of the deductible is met. If the patient has a second eligible medical expense of $3,000, the patient will have to pay $1,000. The $1,000 is the remaining portion of the $5,000 deductible, used in our example that had not been met from the previous $4,000 out of pocket already paid. The remaining $2,000 from the medical bill would be paid according to the terms of the policy. Very likely, the patient would have to pay any co-pay or co-insurance that may be on his plan and all non-eligible charges i.e. pre-existing related if excluded from his policy, and the insurer would pay the balance of eligible charges. Deductibles are amounts customers must pay in addition to any other obligations i.e. premiums, co-pays, co-insurance, non-eligible or non-covered services or charges.

A **co-payment, or co-pay,** is the amount the customer is required to pay in addition to the premiums and after the deductible has been met. Co-pays are common. For example, a patient with a $25 co-pay on in-network primary care physician (PCP) visits and $50 on out of network PCPs goes to their PCP. With few exceptions, the patient will have to pay the co-pay every time they see their PCP even if they have met their deductible. If the PCP charges $150 for the visit, the patient will pay $25 and the insurer may be responsible for the remaining PCP visit charge. It gets a little confusing. The charge may be $150 but the insurer may only "allow" a $100 PCP charge. In such a case, if the PCP is in-network and has agreed to this rate, the "charge" will be $100, and the patient will still owe $25 and the insurer would be responsible for $75. If the PCP is out of network, the patient would be responsible for $50 and the insurer the remaining amount. However, if the PCP charge was $300, and the insurer refuses to pay this amount and only pay a set amount. Let's assume $75. If that were the case, the patient could still be responsible for the remaining $175. That is the $300 charge minus the $50 co-pay that the patient paid minus the $75 the insurance company paid which equals $175. Co-pays are amounts customers must pay in addition to premiums, deductibles, co-insurance or non-eligible or non-covered services or charges.

Co-insurance is a fee, typically stated as a percentage of a charge, the patient is responsible to pay. Assume a patient goes to a PCP and has a $25 co-pay and a 20% co-insurance. If the doctor is in-network and did a procedure that he bills $1000 in addition to his $150 office visit, the patient, or insured, would be required to pay a $25 co-pay to the PCP for the $150 PCP visit and then pay $200 more to the PCP for the patient's 20% portion of the $1,000 bill for the procedure, a total of $225. The insurer would then be responsible for the remaining eligible charges. This is assuming that the deductible has been met. If it has not been met, the patient could be responsible for the full $1,000 for the procedure and could be responsible for the full $150 for the PCP visit. If the PCP is out-of-network, the portion that the patient is responsible for is likely to be even higher i.e. 30%. The co-insurance amount is the amount customers must pay in addition to the insurance premiums, deductibles, co-pays and non-eligible or non-covered services and charges.

Eligible charge is a healthcare expense that the insurance company agrees is covered by the insurance policy. Even if the charge is eligible, it does not guarantee that the insurance company will pay for the charge. It still must meet all the other terms before the insurance company will pay i.e. deductible, co-pays, coinsurance, etc. For example, if a policyholder goes to their PCP and is charged $150 for a visit, it is likely that the insurer will recognize the charge as eligible for coverage. Assuming the deductible has been met and the patient pays the required co-pay of $25 on his policy, the insurer will pay the remaining $125, or whatever the difference is between the insurance negotiated rate between the PCP and insurance company and the amount the patient paid. But if the policyholder goes to a chiropractor or a healer, the insurance company may deem the charge ineligible and pay zero regardless of whether the patient met their deductible or made any payment. In such a case, the policy holder would be responsible for 100% of the charges. It is possible that whatever paid for an ineligible charge may not count towards the deductible amount.

Another reason an insurance company may deem a charge ineligible is that the policy does not cover the service i.e. pre-existing condition not covered under the policy or the treatment is deemed experimental and not covered. A **pre-existing condition** is a condition that the insured has been treated for in the past or exists before the person is covered by the insurer. Insurers may provide coverage but that coverage will not apply to any expenses related to the pre-existing condition. For example, if someone is diagnosed with cancer and applies for health insurance, the insurer will not pay for any expenses related to the cancer. The insurer may pay for expenses related to a skin infection or a car accident but not chemotherapy or anything related to cancer. Even if someone gets treated for pneumonia, the insurer might deny payment arguing that the pneumonia is related to the pre-existing cancer i.e. lung cancer causing "obstructive pneumonia." If the insurance company deems a charge as ineligible, the insurer would pay 0% and the patient would be responsible for 100% of the charge.

Maximum out-of-pocket is meant to be the total amount that a patient would have to pay when one includes deductibles, co-pays and co-insurance. One exception to this may be the policy maximum benefit. If one has a $10,000 maximum out of pocket amount associated with a

$1,000,000.00 maximum policy limit and they are so unfortunate to require an organ transplant or some rare condition for which the treatment exceeds $1,000,000.00, say $2,000,000, the maximum out-of-pocket may not accurately reflect what the patients actual responsibility would be i.e. $1,000,000 in addition to the $10,000 "maximum out of pocket" amount. In addition, should the insurance company deny a charge or service, claim it is not an eligible charge or service, or classify the charge as related to a pre-existing condition that is specifically excluded by the policy language, the patient may be 100% responsible for 100% of the bill regardless of the amount. So even if a customer pays all their premiums, has met their full deductible and pays all co-pays and all co-insurance, the insurance company could theoretically, deny making any payment and the patient would be responsible for the entire charge.

Policy Limit is typically the maximum amount that the insurer will pay towards the eligible healthcare expenses of a policyholder in a specific time period. For example, a $100,000/$500,000 policy limit might mean that there is a $100,000 total limit to the eligible health expenses of the policy holder that the insurer is required to pay in a given year and $500,000 total limit for the policy holder's lifetime. Should an insured patient have a $100,000 policy limit and require major surgery, an organ transplant, treatment for a serious condition or hospitalization that cost $750,000 in a given year, the health insurer would pay up to $100,000 and the patient would be responsible for the remaining $650,000.

In Network and Out-of-Network. This refers to the "providers" of healthcare within the health insurance network. It is important to mention that insurers use the term provider to include any person or entity that provides service to a patient. In the view of insurers, a provider could be a human being such as a physician or a non-physician provider, such as a nurse practitioner, physician assistant, therapist etc. or a business such as a hospital, imaging center or lab. For the purposes of this chapter, the term provider will apply to both human and non-human providers. Otherwise, when I use the term provider, it will refer to physicians and NPPs, not hospitals, laboratories or other non-human entities. In network providers are those who have agreements with the insurer to accept a certain rate for whatever service they may provide to patients with that insurance company's policyholders. Out of network providers are any "provider" that does not have such an agreement with the insurer. The advantage to a patient to receive care from an in-network provider is that the cost to the patient are almost always lower than obtaining care from an out of network provider i.e. lower co-pay or co-insurance. In some instances, an insurer may refuse to pay anything for an out of network provider. The disadvantage to the patient with in-network is that many physicians may refuse to agree to be in-network because the insurer offers very low payments for their service. Thus, sometimes patients have less choice to obtain care for a service or may not be able to see the physician of their choice. Remember all physicians or hospitals are not equal. Some physicians may have better training, experience and reputations. Some physicians and non-physician providers i.e. hospitals, etc. may give better service. Some may have lower complication or infection rates with surgeries, etc. Because insurers are not willing to pay what these out of network providers charge, it limits patients from being able to obtain care from these qualified providers. One could make the argument that a patient can still obtain care from these out of network providers but in order to do so, the patient would have to pay much more and possibly may not be able to afford the extra cost. Sometimes patients must travel farther or obtain care from a provider they are not familiar or comfortable with because the insurance company refuses to pay the preferred providers of the patient that may be local or closer to them.

The advantage for a provider to be in-network is that by agreeing to the fee schedule of the insurers, the provider should get more business. It makes sense. If the insurer will cover more of the costs if the patient chooses an in-network provider, it is more likely that patients will choose in network providers, since it will cost the patients less to do so. Thus, more patients are likely to choose in-network physicians. So, if a physician wants to increase the number of patients who might use his service, even if it is at a lower charge, being in-network could help a physician get more patients. From a business standpoint, it would seem to make sense for all providers to be in network for all insurance companies. The big disadvantage for a provider to be in-network is that the allowed charge is typically much lower than their ordinary and customary charge. So much lower in some cases it may cause the provider to lose money or go out of business. As a result, many providers choose to remain out of network because it makes more financial sense. From the insurer's standpoint, having in-network doctors is advantageous because they can pay less for physician services, increasing potential profits. Another advantage is they can market to the public that they have more in-network physicians to choose from.

The in-network and out-of-network issue, from an insurer or provider's standpoint is understandable. One could make the argument for either side. One could argue that either side is unreasonable. One would think that from a society standpoint, what is, or should be, more important is the patient's perspective. From a patient's standpoint, it makes healthcare more complicated and dilutes the security that health insurance coverage should provide policy holders. The security of knowing that should one get stricken with an illness or disease, they can choose whatever physician or "provider" they wish without a financial penalty.

There are probably circumstances when the insurer or the provider is so unreasonable that the other side cannot agree. For an example, an insurer may pay a physician an amount that does not cover the physician's cost. Perhaps the insurer assumes the physician can make up the losses from other insurers or patients? On the other hand, a physician may demand a fee that 10 times higher than other insurers. There should be a middle ground where reasonable people can agree.

One could make the argument that I have a natural bias favoring the patient and physician. With my degree and knowledge of economics and my experience in business and with negotiations, I can analyze things from a very different perspective than simply as a doctor. In addition, I have worked with insurance leaders and provided professional consulting service to a Fortune 500 insurer which gives me additional knowledge and insight into the insurance industry that many others lack.

It sometimes seems that the more likely reason that the insurer, or the provider, will not agree, or is willing to be flexible, is simply to increase revenue or profits. This seems especially true with the insurers and larger physician and non-physician providers groups i.e. CMGs. Individual physicians and small physician groups who lack significant "size" and resources, often suffer as do patients. Insurers and these large CMGs try to negotiate what is best for themselves and use whatever influence and resources they possess to get their way. They try to use their size and influence with patients and "bully" the other side into agreeing to the terms they want. Because of their large size and enormous financial resources, insurers often get favorable terms to them at the expense of physicians and patients. Even when these CMGs "win" in negotiations, the individual physicians who provide the actual care to the patients do not necessarily benefit. It is possible any gains are kept by the CMG and not passed on to the practicing physicians who treat the patients or the patients themselves. For the sake of what is best for patients and the public, this needs to end. The involved parties need to negotiate in good faith and come to an agreement that will be fair and what is best for patients.

Of course, determining what is fair and who determines what is fair is the tricky part. One could argue appointing a panel, committee or arbitrator to determine what is fair. Sounds simply enough but it is much more complicated. Some things to consider when trying to make it fair:

- Who will appoint the committee or panel members?
- What bias or influence do either side have on who will do the appointing?
- What data will be used to determine a fair price?

- Who will supply this data?
- Who will determine who will supply the data and do they have a bias to either side?
- How will this price be determined?

Such concerns are being raised presently between physicians, physician groups and staffing companies, and insurers regarding "surprise billing" a.k.a. balanced billing, as the two sides both blame the other. Unfortunately, as the two sides argue and give reasons for the other side being the problem, the patient is caught in the middle and continues to suffer.

Insurers should be responsible to make sure consumers understand insurance policies and what the insurance company is selling them

I do not have an issue with insurance companies offering many different products with various deductibles amounts, co-pay amounts, co-insurance amounts, policy limit amounts, etc. In a sense, I applaud them for providing choice to consumers. Choice is usually a good thing so long as one fully understands the pros and cons of the choices. Where I have an issue, and where the public and government should be concerned, is that it confuses the public. The insurers do not make sure the public understands the policies, and because of this, people may select insurance plans that are harmful to them.

Insurance companies have, or should have, an obligation to make sure their policy holders understand the health insurance policies that the public is paying for. Insurers need to assure that the people understand the policies that are intended to protect them, should the need arise, before the public buys it. Many people do not fully understand what coverage they have or the deficiencies of the coverage they have until they have a significant health expense or medical emergency and often that is too late.

Ask most anyone and many will say health is important. Given the importance of health and healthcare to our country and of having a healthy population, it is worth mentioning again that insurers should be responsible to make sure consumers understand insurance policies and what the insurance company is selling them. There should be little to no confusion whatsoever to the consumer, about what the policy covers, what it does not cover, any amounts and how much the insured must pay. If given a scenario, the customer should easily be able to determine how much the insurer will pay and how much the insured will have to pay. Keep it simple. If it is not this simple, then the insurance company needs to make it simpler until it is. If the insurer is not able or willing to do so, then perhaps the insurer should not be allowed to sell insurance to the public or at a minimum, be held accountable financially.

We are talking about the health of our citizens and the health of our friends and families. This is very important; insurers need to stop making excuses and just fix it. If they can't make it so simple that someone with a 5th grade education can understand, then we have a problem. People with college degrees don't understand their policies. One must wonder if the system is intentionally this confusing and complicated. Why? Insurance companies have lots of resources and there are some things that would be easy to do to help simplify things but are not done. Something as simple as printing a patient's deductible amount on their insurance card would easily help people know how much they must pay before the insurer pays a penny. Why isn't this done by all insurers? Many insurance cards fail to have deductible amounts printed on them. It's hard to imagine that with all the money insurers have and the people on their payroll that no one has thought of something so simple that would remove confusion and prevent lots of wasted time. Do the insurers not do this because they don't want the insured to know the truth and be upset? Do the insurers intentionally try to keep consumers uninformed? If the customer knew what poor coverage the insurer sold them, the consumer might get upset, complain to regulators, choose another insurer, decide on alternatives to insurance or not buy insurance at all.

The way insurance companies sell insurance is unfair to the patient and one can argue an unethical way of doing business

Perhaps there should be some independent group, agency or panel that surveys the public and asks specifics about the insurance plans. This panel could be elected officials or appointed by a state's Supreme Court in hopes of minimizing bias. If the insured score below a certain score, the insurer could be penalized. I am not a big advocate of lots of government regulations but perhaps that is one consideration for something of this importance. Perhaps this will motivate insurers to not make excuses but instead to come up with some simple and easy to understand solutions to the many problems with the current system. Perhaps this should be a licensing requirement? The insurer should be responsible that the customer understands what the insurer is selling to the consumer. Remember, it should be so simple that a 5th grader could understand it.

One excuse the insurers might say is that the insured can call us anytime with a question. Sounds nice but, this is just another obstacle.

- This is often time consuming; there can be delays before speaking to someone.
- The insurance representative will want information to verify identity etc. and this takes more time.
- The insurance representative sometimes gives the wrong or confusing information. The representative may use common statements, read from a script or speak in a confusing manner, but may not actually answer the question that the consumer has.
- There are times when the representative may tell the insured that the provider or other facility will explain.

People don't have time to waste; they have many responsibilities such as family, work, friends, church, etc. They may not have the extra time to call and wait and be frustrated during insurance company determined hours. Thus, they may not call because they know they don't have the time or because of the hassles they might encounter. If they don't, the customer suffers, not the insurer. The insurer is likely better off because it may not have to pay for care that the customer may need but does not receive. The point: the current system seems less focused on the things that matter to the patient, convenience or care; it is not efficient or effective and has many obstacles for the consumer to effectively and conveniently get the information they need in order to fully understand the insurance policies or get the care they may require. It seems designed to benefit the insurance company and not the patient, consumer or public. Given how much people pay for health insurance and how much insurance companies make in revenue, one would think that the public would get a better product and better service. The burden of making sure the public understands needs to rest on the insurer.

The insurance company gets paid upfront by the consumer before care is ever provided, whether treatment is needed or not

Another issue with the current healthcare system is insurance companies complicate matters by requiring physicians and other healthcare providers to do things that should be done by the insurer. It would be much easier for the insured patient, if the insurance company handled matters related to insurance. Insurers should be responsible for paying the full amount due to the physician and other non-physician providers that include all co-insurance, co-pays and deductibles. The insurance company would then collect these from their insured. This way, in their time of need, patients only need to be concern themselves with their health and not be distracted with insurance related issues. The current healthcare system requires others to enforce the terms that the insurance company developed and sold to the consumer. This is usually often done at the time the patient requires care. The insurer is the one who sold the policy to the public. The insurer is the one that wrote the policy. The insurer is the one who has the contractual arrangement with the policy holder. The insurer is the one who collects premiums from the insured. Doesn't it make the most sense to make the insurer collect any required money or payments from the patient? It is not fair to the patient to make non-insurance people responsible to enforce what the insurer sold.

Sell something and then let others deal with the mess

It does not seem fair that physicians, physician representatives, hospital representatives, imaging center representatives, laboratory representative or anyone else, beside the insurer, should have to explain to the patient what the policy that was sold by the insurer, covers or does not cover. The way insurance companies sell insurance is unfair to the patient and one can argue an unethical way of doing business. Sell something and then let others deal with the mess. Let others help consumers understand what the insurers did not explain well enough. Let others have the task of telling patients what they don't want to hear. Let others, not the insurer who wrote the policy, explain what their insurance does not cover, or requires from the patient. Perhaps the insurers know that a certain percentage of insured people can't or won't pay co-pays, co-insurance or deductibles and want the doctors, hospitals or others getting stuck not getting paid? If so, it seems unethical and should be illegal. This could be a way for the insurance company to increase its profits even more. Perhaps the insurance company wants the doctors or hospitals to look like the bad guys trying to collect money from the patient even after they have "paid" money at the time of service instead of the insurer being viewed as the bad guy. The insurer gets paid upfront by the consumer before care is ever provided, whether treatment is needed or not. By requiring the insurer to pay all fees and amounts required of the insurer and the patient directly to doctors, hospitals and other non-physician providers and then getting reimbursed by the policy holder that they sold the policy to seems to be the simplest, easiest, most transparent and fairest for the patient and the public.

72 million Americans have medical bill problems or are paying off medical debt[28]

Another concerning matter regarding health insurance policies that insurance companies are selling to the public is that they have the potential to financially ruin families. According to information presented at the 2019 American College of Emergency Physicians (ACEP) Leadership Advocacy Conference (LAC) in Washington DC, the average family in America has $700 in emergency cash and $6000 in family savings yet a typical health insurance plan has a $7000 deductible.[29] Search online and many sites and sources indicate that any unexpected or emergency expense over $600 or even $400 can cause financial hardship to many Americans. For many things, including emergency room visits, the patient typically must pay 100% of the deductible before the insurance company will pay a penny. In the event someone has a medical emergency in which the treatment costs $6,000 or more, the family's entire savings will be wiped out. By the time the deductible of $7000 is reached, the family is already underwater $1,000 and after that, the family still must pay co-pays or co-insurance and other non-covered expenses. With the costs of healthcare today, it does not take much to have a $7,000 bill. One emergency room visit, evaluation and treatment can easily exceed $6000. Nearly 1 in 5 of all Americans have medical debt in collections.[30] According to a Commonwealth Fund survey, as many as 2 in 5 working Americans (72 million) have medical bill problems or are paying off medical debt.[31]

Let's now discuss the point that insurers may be selling something that may be worse than no insurance at all. In the above example, insurers may collect $500 or $1,000 a month in insurance premiums. For family plans, monthly premium amounts may far exceed $1,000. Let's assume somewhere in the middle, $750/month or $9,000 for the year. Let's assume an ER visit costs $7000. Someone who may need emergency care may realize that their visit could be expensive and if they understand what their policy with a $7000 deductible means, choose not to seek necessary emergency care because they can't afford to pay for it and don't want to put their family in financial ruins. So, the policy that is supposed to protect the public by spreading out risk, doesn't properly spread out any risk or provide protection. In this example, even though the patient bought an expensive $9,000 health insurance policy, it doesn't provide any protection from the $7,000 costs. The patient is paying a lot of money but does not benefit from having it; the patient would have to pay the entire $7000 out of pocket. The end-result is that the patient does not get care. In such a situation, it would be better if the patient had no insurance. A person who pays $9,000 a year in insurance premiums for a policy that has a $7,000 deductible will be responsible to pay $16,000 before the insurance company will pay a penny. If the patient did not have insurance, the patient would be able to save the $9000 paid in annual premiums and use it to pay cash for the entire $7,000 without having to deplete the family savings and risking bankruptcy and all the negatives that go with it. In such a case, the patient would still have $2,000 to use for healthcare, pay down debt or to save for the future.

One would think that the government would step in and investigate this or even penalize the insurance carriers selling such policies. The argument is that insurers know, or should know, that the average family only has an average of $700 in emergency cash and an average of $6000 in savings. The insurers know or should know that selling an insurance policy with a $7000 deductible could be detrimental to or destroy a family with limited resources. Thus, one could argue that the insurers should be penalized and forced to pay for all healthcare costs, or at least much more than the "inadequate policy" covers that the consumer was sold.

A similar argument was made after the housing crisis and financial crisis that followed. Mortgage lenders were criticized for making mortgages to borrowers that the lenders knew, or should have known, borrowers were unable to afford. Even though borrowers signed the paperwork with many disclosures that the mortgage lenders created, many believed that the borrowers did not understand the terms of the mortgage. The lenders were held accountable for their part in the housing crisis and were required to pay tens of billions of dollars in fines and penalties for their poor behavior and involvement that caused the housing meltdown and financial crisis that resulted. Why are healthcare contracts any different?

As stated at the beginning of Chapter 2, insurers spread risk. Health insurers lose money on some people i.e. the costs to the insurance company to pay for covered treatments and care exceeds the policy premiums the person pays i.e. high healthcare users with frequent and expensive healthcare needs. In addition, there are other costs the insurer must pay such as salaries to its employees, rent, taxes, etc. but you get the idea. Before you feel sorry for insurance companies, don't. Health insurance companies make billions upon billions of dollars each year in profits. While they may lose money on a person here or there i.e. high healthcare users, they make plenty of money from other insured people who don't use much healthcare i.e. low healthcare users that pay premiums far in excess of what they use. So essentially these low healthcare users, who choose to buy insurance, help subsidize the care of others who use more healthcare than their premiums cover. This is the concept of spreading risk amongst large groups of people. The people who do not require much care and pay more in premiums than they use in healthcare expenses, subsidize the costs of healthcare for those who pay less in premiums than they use in healthcare expenses.

In Obamacare, low healthcare users are forced to subsidize higher healthcare users. They had no choice

Remember the Affordable Care Act (ACA), often referred to as

"Obamacare?" The ACA was signed into law by President Barack Obama on March 23, 2010. Part of the ACA requires everyone, with few exceptions, to have health insurance. If someone did not have health insurance, that person would be required to pay a financial penalty. Sounds kind of crazy huh. You must pay money for the right to not have something. Ever wonder why it required everyone to carry healthcare or pay a penalty? The idea is to make everyone carry insurance including those who may ordinarily choose not to. By doing so, there will likely be more people paying premiums (or penalties) that are low healthcare users. These people would essentially help subsidize the insurance for high users of healthcare and those who did not pay personally for their insurance. Some people, unless forced, may choose not to buy health insurance because they are healthy and realize they are likely to pay much more in health insurance premiums than what they would spend paying for any healthcare out of pocket. People who decide not to buy insurance are essentially taking on the risk themselves. They would benefit if they are correct and likely have high bills and potentially go bankrupt if they are wrong. In Obamacare, these people are forced to buy health insurance, or pay a premium, that will help fund the losses caused by others who are insured and using more in healthcare dollars than they pay in premiums. While private insurance uses this strategy of using money making policies to subsidize money losing policies, the consumer has the choice to buy health insurance or not buy insurance from an insurance company. Put another way, in the ACA model, low healthcare users are forced to subsidize higher healthcare users. They have no choice. This is one of the biggest criticisms of the ACA.

Earlier in this chapter, I mentioned that insurance companies serve as a watchdog over many within the healthcare system and discussed how this could potentially help keep healthcare costs down. "Why Your Health Insurer Doesn't Care About Your Big Bills" by Marshall Allen brings up a great point why this may not be the case and why it may be in the insurance company's interest not to keep costs down. In what might be considered an attempt to limit the profits of insurance companies, the ACA included something that is referred to as the 80/20 rule or the medical loss ratio (MLR). The 80/20 rule requires that at least 80 cents of every dollar paid in premiums to the insurer must be spent by the insurance company on medical costs or quality improvement activities. For larger insured groups, the ratio is 85:15 (85/15). The remaining 15-20%, can be used for other expenses such as overhead, marketing and profits. While on the surface, this sounds like a reasonable method to limit profits and encourage money to be spent on policy holders and may be the intention of the law, it may contribute to higher health care costs. This is referred to as a "perverse incentive."[32] If we assume an insurance company makes a 3% profit after all medical, quality improvement activity, marketing, overhead and all other expenses are paid, then assuming overhead costs remained constant, the insurer would make more profits if the medical expenses went up. Allen uses the following example to illustrate his point:

> "It's as if a mom told her son he could have 3 percent of a bowl of ice cream. A clever child would say, 'make it a bigger bowl'"[33]

The higher the medical costs and quality improvement expenses, assuming constant overhead costs, the more potential dollar amount in profits that an insurer can make. Assuming a constant overhead, for every 4-dollar increase in medical costs, an extra dollar can go towards insurance company profits. The insurer may have a perverse incentive to want or allow medical expenses to increase. This would seem to conflict with the insurer serving as a watchdog and keeping healthcare prices low.

So how do we make things such that insurance companies change their behavior and act in ways that will help provide lower costs and result in better healthcare? In the next chapter, I will discuss three possible solutions that have the potential to improve coverage, increase access, increase available options, lower rates and bring peace of mind and security to the public.

Chapter 3 Talking Points:

- The purpose of insurance is to spread risk in order to help protect the public i.e. security and peace of mind
- Employer sponsored health insurance policies cover about 152,000,000 people and costs approximately $7000 for single coverage plans and $20,000 for family coverage plans
- Insurance premiums have risen at a much faster rate than either employee wages or inflation.
- Amounts people pay in deductibles on employer sponsored insurance plans have increased by more than 50% in the past 5 years and over 60% of workers must pay a co-payment, and about a 25% co-insurance, when they see a primary care physician or a specialist.
- Many people do not understand the insurance plans they are sold or how much they will have to pay when they receive treatment i.e. How much do you have to pay if you go to the ER and the ER charges are $12,000?
- Insurers should have the responsibility to make sure the public fully understands the policies people are being sold before they buy it.

Edward Shaheen, M.D.

Chapter Four:
POSSIBLE SOLUTIONS TO THE HEALTH INSURANCE PROBLEM

Increase Competition

Current laws and regulations limit the ease in which insurance can be offered. Many insurance companies exist but not all of them offer health insurance in all states or in all regions of all states. There are reports of certain areas where there may only be one licensed insurer offering health insurance. As one might imagine, this limits the choices and often results in higher premiums. Competition on the other hand, often causes competitors to lower prices in order to attract potential customers. In addition, the competing insurers may offer more options, better coverage and other perks to induce the public to choose their company over a competitor.

Many argue the free market is not working. I caution anyone who believes this to hold their judgment until a free market truly exists

Why are there markets where there may only be one or two insurers offering health insurance? Such situations are primed for insurers to take advantage of the public. This may explain the exploding costs of health insurance in many areas. When there is only one insurer, that insurer essentially has monopoly power. If a consumer wants health insurance, they must buy it from that one insurer. This is ridiculous and should not be tolerated. Legislators need to stop catering to insurance lobbyists and put the people first. They need to pass legislation allowing any qualified insurer to offer their products in any state. It's PK to allow competition and the free market to work. Many argue the free market is not working. I caution anyone who believes this to hold their judgment until we allow a free market to truly exist. When these barriers are implemented by legislation, these artificial barriers do not allow a free market to exist. Give us a reasonably free market and let it work; while it may not be perfect, I believe it will work much better than the current broken system we have.

Lifetime Health Insurance Policies

We have some understanding of what is important to insurance companies and how they make money. The more people they cover and the more premiums they collect, the more money they will take in. The less they pay out in claims, by denying specialty referrals, testing, imaging and other services, the more they can delay payments, and the less services people use, the more potential profits they can make. Maximizing profits and delivering good investment returns to their investors is how insurers keep their shareholders happy. Their primary objective does not align with keeping people healthy or providing easy access to medical evaluation and treatment.

Some argue that insurers have too much influence over lawmakers. They may have a point. Insurers are amongst the largest companies in the world and have an army of paid lobbyists to promote their cause, often at odds with what is best for the public and the people who provide services to the public. Insurers are amongst the biggest contributors to politicians and political groups. In 2018, the insurance industry spend over $150 million on lobbying.[34] While politicians should not be influenced by contributions, the large sums spent on lobbying legislators certainly has the appearance of influencing what laws are written, go to a vote and how politicians cast their votes on such legislation. Perhaps the public should demand reform of our political system, but that is for another discussion and time. The point is to bring up some of the challenges we face adopting laws that benefit the public and perhaps explain why something that seems to be common sense, has not already occurred.

Another way to improve the current insurance problem would be to require any insurer who offers health insurance coverage to commit to coverage for a longer period of time without the insurance company being able to cancel the policy as long as premiums are paid. Perhaps a minimum of 10 years, 20 years or even life coverage and being required to commit upfront to what the costs of the insurance will be each year. Lifetime coverage seems to be the optimal time period for the public so we will focus our discussion on lifetime coverage. The idea is the longer the time period, the more protected the public will be. This should eliminate surprise price increases that can bankrupt or force families to choose to go without health insurance. Perhaps having the premium increases limited to a reasonable cost of living index i.e. consumer price index (CPI) is a fairer way of determining rate increase amounts. Doing this should immediately slow the rate of price increases to healthcare. In recent decades, health insurance premiums have far outpaced the rate of wage increases and inflation. Lifetime coverage and tying premium rate increases to the CPI would protect the insured and public from surprise price increases that makes health insurance unaffordable to so many.

Typically, after evaluating your information and determining your "risk," the insurer will decide if it will offer coverage and will quote a premium for such coverage. The coverage is typically an annual cost broken down into monthly costs. The problem is if the insurer determines that a person is no longer "worthy" of coverage for whatever reason (they lost money covering the insured, the insured became sick and used healthcare resources above what the insurer felt was reasonable or financially advantageous to the insurer or that the insurer may lose money on a policy in the future), the insurer may deny the person coverage or significantly raise the premium when it comes time to renew the policy. This is not good for the public nor does it help make healthcare better. This lack of predictability makes it worse for the consumer, the public and society. If the insurer does not cancel, they can raise the premium on coverage. It may be a small rise in price, it may be a high rise in price. The problem is the consumer doesn't know if the insurer will raise prices or by how much and whether they will be able to afford it after the price increase. Hence, this unknown puts the insured and their family's health and well-being in jeopardy. The current broken healthcare system does not provide the public with the proper security and safety net.

If the goal of healthcare is to make people healthy and keep them healthy, especially in the long term, we need to assure people that we are committed to doing so for the long term. Considering the huge amounts of money that insurers make, it is reasonable to expect insurers to make the public's health a priority and to assume more risk. Currently, if an insurer decides your risk and is wrong, they are relatively safe. They are only on the hook for a year, after which they can decide to raise your premium or not renew your policy. The person is then stuck without insurance or must look for another insurer. Instead of shifting more and more risk to the consumer, as insurers have been doing, we need to shift more risk back to the insurer. Isn't this the whole idea behind insurance to begin with? It should spread risk away from the individual. By making it a requirement for insurers to offer health insurance for life and to state what the rate will be each year, the public can feel secure and confident that so long as they pay the pre-set premium, they will have health insurance and the ability to get necessary healthcare and treatment as needed. Removing uncertainty and protecting the public will help make healthcare easier to understand should improve the health of patients.

This concept of lifelong health insurance policies makes sense

In addition to offering predictability and affordability, this requirement does something else that is important. It aligns the insurer's goal with the public's best interest. In the current system, insurers evaluate a person's information and decide on how much they think it will cost them to provide that person with health insurance coverage. They then have a formula that includes healthcare expenses, other costs (administrative, operations, etc.) and give a premium that typically has a cushion to cover for a margin of error and profits. If they are right or over estimated costs, they make profits or higher profits than expected. In such cases, do they lower the insurance premiums? They should but they typically don't. Insurers will continue to offer coverage if the insurer expects to make money from the insured over time. But should the consumer have the misfortune of becoming ill or developing a chronic condition or terminal illness, the insurer can jack up the premium or dump the insured come renewal time. This arrangement is not in the insured consumer's, or public's best interest. It seems to be skewed in the insurance company's best interest.

By requiring insurers to cover their insured for life, then the insurer can no longer do this. They will have to continue to cover the insured person's healthcare expenses. Instead of simply trying to make money in the short term based on year to year costs and utilization, they will have a big financial incentive to keep people healthy. That's right, insurers will still want to maximize profits, but they will do so by keeping people healthy. They will know they cannot cancel a policy so they will have to become more engaged, aligned and incentivized to keep the insured healthy now and for the long term. By doing so, the lifetime expenses will be minimized, and their potential profits will be maximized. A "win-win" situation. With the current system, it seems that if the customer wins, the insurer is more likely to lose and vice versa.

By changing insurance in this way, instead of withholding authorization for certain testing or evaluations, denial of treatments or other decisions that currently benefit their bottom line, the insurers may become an advocate for the public. The insurer may help increase access and allow a patient to be seen sooner or have preventative testing or treatment and willing to pay for it knowing that by doing so, its short term expenses may be higher but in the long run, its costs will be reduced and profits maximized. They would no longer be able to make people wait and then cancel policies upon renewal before they must pay for the costs of the procedures, testing or evaluations that they denied while policies were still in place. Under the current system if an insurer refuses to renew a policy or raises rates so much that someone cannot afford it, then the customer will have to fight with the next insurer in hopes that they will approve and pay for these services. Of course, the next policy will likely be much more expensive than the last policy assuming the next insurer will agree to provide health insurance to the consumer.

This concept of lifelong health insurance policies with no expiration makes sense. It reverses some of the problems with the current broken system. First, the insurer will no longer put short-term profits ahead of the consumer (it appears that insurers sometimes forget to take into consideration the concept of shared risk and who insurance is supposed to help). Insurers may lose money on some consumers, but they will more than make it up on other consumers. The reasoning for allowing insurance companies to exist and operate should be to provide a valuable and needed service to the public, spread risk, protect the public and makes society better off. It is not for the purpose of allowing insurance companies to make tens of billions of dollars annually. Trying to make money on each covered person removes this inherent protection of people's ability to access and obtain quality care for illnesses and injuries that can occur. Dropping the person gives the impression that the insurer only cares about the money. The insurer is happy to cover and "protect" the consumer from high healthcare expenses when the consumer doesn't need care but once the consumer does need care, insurers want to unload the consumer because insurers' primary goal is not the consumer's best long-term health, it is profits. Providing lifetime health coverage will align the public's best interest with insurance company's motivation of making profits for its shareholders. It is important to say, there is nothing wrong with making profits. We want insurers to be profitable and financially sound so they can continue to provide the public with a valuable service. Freedom of markets and capitalism, particularly "benevolent capitalism," is a great incubator of thought, ideas, innovation and advancements that help mankind. We should make sure that it functions in a fair and healthy way for society.

Second, lifetime health insurance would benefit the reputation of insurers. Many have a very low opinion of insurers. Ask members of the public, health care providers and patients, many have a very low opinion of them. In fairness to insurers, some of what they do is reasonable, and they play a very important role in healthcare. To the insurers' credit, part of the reason why they are so hated by some may be because they are so good at what they do. They try to maximize profits and by doing so, they cause harm to others. They use their influence, money and power to their advantage which is not necessarily in the best interest of the public. In fact, often their best interest may be at direct odds to the best interests of others. By requiring insurers to provide lifetime health insurance coverage and aligning their goals with the goal of making healthcare better for patients, we may be able to convert their success of getting their way, influencing politicians and making obscene profits into better healthcare to the public and society. If done properly, insurers can still make lots of money and allow a better healthcare system to exist. If insurers were aligned and their goals aligned with society's goal of fixing our broken healthcare system, the insurers could improve their image and become more respected and liked. In a sense, insurers could be their own watchdogs in addition to any other oversight. Instead of others trying to force them to do the right thing for the public, insurers will do this themselves. Since the best interests of the public and the insurers will be closely aligned, by doing what is best for themselves will likely be what is best for the consumer, and vice versa. It will make good business sense and maximize the insurer's long-term profits.

There are potential drawbacks to this model of requiring healthcare until death. If one considers only money and takes a dark or sinister view of insurers, one might wonder whether the insurer would deny evaluations or treatments to those who were high users of healthcare and the most expensive to cover. Not to accuse anyone or any company, but from a purely financial standpoint, there might be incentive to withhold evaluation or treatments and allow high cost, insured patients to die. Of course, it would be unethical and very possibly illegal and there could be liability exposure should an insurer take this route, but it is something worth mentioning. If an insurer evaluates an insured and realizes that the insurer is paying a significant amount in healthcare costs and the patient is unlikely to get better, the insurer is stuck. Because this model does not allow the insurer to deny or cancel renewal after the policy is first issued unless premiums are not paid and does not allow price increases beyond what is stated upfront when the policy is originally written, the insurer is stuck. They would not be able to cancel the policy or not renew the policy as they are able to do now. They would be able to increase the cost of the policy but only to the extent that was agreed when the policy was first written i.e. increases based on CPI. Unlike now, when an insurer can increase rates by huge amounts from year to year. Some, particularly insurers, may argue this model is unfair and would put the stability of insurers and safety of the public in jeopardy. A response might be that the current system is broken and is failing right before us. Many people are unable to afford health insurance; people with health insurance coverage often cannot afford to use it; the healthcare costs in our country is the highest in the world yet our healthcare is far from the best.

In addition, insurers should be experts at insurance. They typically are the ones who have the data, have been in the business for decades and the people who write the policies. Collectively, insurers are billionaires. They have shifted more and more risk and costs onto the insured; the people that we should be most concerned about and the people that insurance is intended to protect. It is time that the risk is shifted back to the insurers. If they want to continue to do business with the public, they will have to take more risks. If they can do their job well and make accurate predictions through actuarial data and taking into consideration the many factors associated with healthcare, then they should continue to make billions of dollars. If not, perhaps they need to step aside and allow newer companies to provide needed services at a better value and with better results. Insurers need to have more accountability. If we allow the free market to work, there will be others who enter the market who are willing to do so.

Currently, if the insurers are good at what they do and predict correctly, they will make handsome profits and be sustainable over time. If the insurers are wrong and poor at predicting or handling their role in healthcare, they simply raise rates and still make money. This may be a great system for the insurers, but it is a broken way of doing things for society. If insurers are not good at predicting costs and performing their role in healthcare, perhaps they need to be allowed to lose money and go out of business. Some may argue that we cannot let insurers go out of business because it will hurt the public. I disagree. Allowing insurers who do not know what they are doing and or who cannot protect the public without fleecing them is unacceptable. Create a free market that allows competition and allow "survival of the fittest" to take its course. Nurture and encourage benevolent capitalism and allow the free market to work. Companies that do not meet the needs or the demands of their customers should be allowed to fail. Such companies often bring little value and may erode the confidence and security of the public. Better run and performing insurers will rise and become the new leaders who can do a better job keeping people secure and healthy at a lower cost and help make people and society better off than it is today. Government needs to pass legislation that will allow competition to flourish and encourage better options and models to help make healthcare better for the public and help the people that they are supposed to serve. If government fails to do so, the people need to voice their opinion and, if necessary, exercise their power at the ballot box to ensure that government is held accountable to create an environment where free markets can work, and competition is nurtured.

Health/Life Insurance Hybrid

This model would require insurers to offer combined lifelong health and life insurance policies to all covered persons. This added twist should help ease concerns about a potential drawback that was mentioned in the lifetime healthcare model. This would encourage insurers to operate in a manner that would improve healthcare, by incentivizing insurers to do what is most likely to keep people healthy in the long term. While it may increase utilization in the short term by increasing and encouraging access when evaluation and care is felt to be needed, it would improve the health of the insured. This is good for improving healthcare and will help society. It also would discourage insurers from denying approvals or payments for evaluations by a physician or non-physician provider, laboratory tests, imaging, therapy or other treatments, which many believe occurs too frequently in the current system.

The logic behind this model is to encourage insurers not to deny services or other healthcare needs but instead to encourage all tests and services to be done in order to keep people healthy in the long term. By doing so, the insurers would save money by avoiding having to pay out high dollar amounts in life insurance prematurely. To understand this, we must first understand a little about how life insurance policies works.

Life insurance is like health, or most any other type of insurance. It spreads risk and relies heavily on statistics. A customer's information is obtained, along with insurer's historical and actuarial data. This information and data are analyzed, and risk is determined, and a value is assigned. This value is based on the risk, likelihood of something happening or not and the cost of various things, that may be necessary. Once done, a premium is assigned that includes all expected costs associated along with a profit margin for the insurer which might also include a margin for error.

Whole life insurance can be 5-10 times more expensive than term life insurance

Life insurance companies make money by collecting insurance premiums and making investment income from that premium money. If this totals more than they pay out to the families of the insured, or whomever is named as the beneficiary of the policy and the insurer's associated expenses, the life insurance companies are profitable. Based on life expectancies of the person which is estimated by the insurance company based on many factors that may include various factors such as the person's age, current health status, medical history, family history, tobacco use or abstinence, line of work, etc. and the amount of the policy payout at time of death, the insurance company can calculate an estimated cost of that particular policy.

Life insurance companies make a lot of money. They charge premiums each month or year and continue to collect until the policy ends or the insured dies. Not all insurance policies pay out benefits. In fact, most term life insurance policies pay nothing to the customer or his/her beneficiaries. The customer pays premiums every year for 10, 20 or more years and no one gets a payout; the insurance company collects all those premiums and gets free use of the money collected and the money made from investing it. Typically, the person will select an amount of the policy benefit; the amount that the insurer agrees to pay his/her estate or the beneficiary that the insured names. Since the insured, by definition and terms of the policy, will be dead when the policy is paid, the insured will not receive the benefit. His or her estate will or whomever the insured decides to benefit from the policy. Understand that insurance companies have other costs associated with doing business other than just the payout such as sales, marketing, staff, rent, taxes and other expenses. For the purposes of this example and simple explanation, we will not mention over and over when discussing costs to insurer and primarily focus on premiums and policy payout to keep things simple. We will assume these other costs that insurers incur as part of doing business are included in "policy payout."

Sometimes life insurance premiums alone are not enough to cover a payout amount of a life insurance policy. Even with this shortfall, life insurance companies are still able to still make money. Life insurers use the money they receive in policy premiums essentially for free until they must pay out a policy claim when an insured person dies. This is where the insurance company often makes most of its money from a life insurance policy. This may sound boring but the power of compounding interest or investing and reinvesting gains is impressive. In fact, we will see that if the insurer relied only on policy premiums alone without taking into consideration other revenue that can be generated from that money, the insurer would lose money.

There are different forms of cash value life insurance, the best known called whole life insurance. For the purposes of this book, we will use whole life as the example of cash value life insurance and compare it to term life insurance. For example. Let's use a 20-year-old male as an example. If he wished to obtain life insurance to protect his wife and or family, he could choose to get term life or cash value life insurance. According to policygenius.com website, he would pay $15.90 per month, for a 20-year term life insurance $250,000.00 policy.[35] So long as he paid his premiums, if he were to die within the 20-year time frame in which the policy covers, his beneficiary would be paid the $250,000. For a woman, the policy premium would be less. The premiums are calculated based on formulas used to determine risks and women, all other things being equal, are less likely to die during a 20-year policy period than a man. For a whole life policy of $100,000.00 for the same 20-year-old man, the policy premium would be $85.45[36] per month forever. That's not a typo, whole life would cost 5-6 times more for less coverage ($100,000 vs. $250,000). It is estimated that whole life insurance typically costs 6-10 times more than term life.[37] So long as the policyholder paid premiums each month, the policy would remain in effect until death and the $100,000 would be paid upon his death to whatever beneficiary the policyholder designated as the beneficiary in the policy. It is suggested to speak with a trusted insurance expert if you would like to learn the specifics of and the pros and cons of each type of life insurance.

In term life, the premiums are much less expensive and easier for people to afford. The drawback is that these policies expire after their "term" and even though you might pay each month for 20 years, you will not be insured after the 20 years and the policy will not have any value. But the idea is that in 20 years, one may be in a better financial position and no longer need life insurance i.e. no longer has young dependent children or now has more assets and savings. Essentially, the insurance company takes in all the policy payments and will pay out zero so long as the insured is still alive after 20 years. If one wishes to maintain life insurance, he will have to get another policy which would be more expensive because he would be 20 years older. A 40-year-old man would pay on average $21.75 per month, a 50-year-old $47.86 per month for a 20-year term life insurance policy. With whole life, it does not expire and does have some value that you can redeem after you have paid so many premium payments. Whole life may also have some other benefits for some people. The bad news is that whole life is very expensive compared to term-life and one should fully understand the different types of life insurance before deciding which type to buy. According to talk show and radio personality Dave Ramsey, whole life policies can cost as much as 20 times as much as a term life policy for the same amount of coverage.[38] He is quite critical of whole life insurance even calling whole life "crap" and refers to whole life as "the payday lender of the middle class."[39] Many people who buy whole life, often cancel or allow policies to expire due to the costs. According to policygenius.com, the cost for a 40-year-old man for whole life is $196.25 per month for a $100,000 policy (compared to $21.75 per month for a $250,000 term life policy) and $233.94 per month for $100,000 whole life policy for a 50-year-old man (compared to $47.86 per month for a $250,000 term life policy). A lot more money for a lot less policy face value amount or benefit.

Assume the insured has a $250,000 term-life policy lives until the age of 80 years old. At that time, the insurer would pay nothing to the term life holder since the policy would have expired at age 40 and would have no value since he "outlived the term" of the policy. Assuming policy holder paid each month for the 20 years, he would have paid a total of $3,816 ($15.90/mo. X 12 months per year X 20 years) and neither he nor any beneficiary would receive any payout benefits from the term policy. So, the life insurer has a potential profit of $3,816 plus whatever the insurance company could make using the premiums collected over the 20 years and beyond. Of course, there are some costs of mailing, administrative and other expenses. Of course, there are the rare cases when someone does die unexpectedly and there will be a policy payout of $250,000. The vast majority of twenty-year-olds with life insurance live beyond forty. Their premiums, and the income generated from those premiums, far exceed the payouts for the rare death that might occur in younger insured policyholders. This is obviously rare, otherwise the life insurers would not be able to stay in business.

Now, assume the same 80-year-old had a $100,000 whole life policy since age 20, and paid the premium of $85.45 each month for 60 years, he would have paid a total of $61,524 ($85.45 X 12 X 60) in policy premiums. If he started the whole life policy at age 30, 40 and 50 and lived until age 80, he would have paid a total of $73,320, $94,200 and $84,218.40 respectively. So long as the insured pays the premium, the beneficiary will be paid the $100,000 policy amount upon death. Unlike term life where beneficiary seldom gets benefits because the insured outlives the term of the policy, whole life plans will pay benefits every time so long as the policy conditions are met. One might ask, how can insurers afford to do this and stay in business? The payout is more than the total of collected premiums in all cases. If the insurer relied only on policy premiums alone to make money, they would lose money. But when you take into consideration the insurer is able to collect the premiums each month for 30, 40 or 50 years and invest this money, sometimes making an 8-12% annual return on their investments, you can begin to understand why life insurance is quite profitable for the life insurance companies.

As a rule, if one divides 70 by the annual rate of return on an investment, the quotient will be the approximate number of years it will take for the amount to double. The rule is not perfect but is a good approximation. If one assumes that life insurance companies invest in the stock market and only get a modest average annual return of 7% over time, the amount will double about every 10 years. This a conservative return as the average annual return before inflation in the stock market (S&P 500) over the last century is about 10%.[40] Every 10 years, the amount will double again. So, if an insurer invests $1 and gets an average annual return of 7% over time, in 60 years that original $1 will be worth approximately $64. This demonstrates the power of compounding returns. If we use the premium policy example of $85.45 per month, the insurer will collect about $1,025 in just the first year. If the insurer invests that $1,025 instead of the $1, we used in the example, after 60 years, the insurer will have $65,600. Remember, this is only the first year of a policy premium invested over 60 years. This amount does not take into consideration the $1,025 in collected premiums from year 2 invested for 59 years, year 3 invested for 58 years, year 4 invested for 57 years and so on until year 59. The collected premiums, along with the investment proceeds, is often in the hundreds of thousands of dollars or more for a $100,000 policy. If the policyholder stops paying or cancels, because it is too expensive or for other reason, then the policy is no longer in effect and there will be no payment to any beneficiary. "All" of the policy premiums collected, along with the money made from investing the policy premiums, is profits. This may not be 100% accurate as whole life plans have a small portion of the premium that acts to build value to the insured and the insurer does have overhead expenses that it must pay. Without getting too complicated, there may be some exceptions, but the example illustrates the high profit potential in the life insurance business. There is a lot of money in life insurance so long as one knows what they are doing, and actual outcomes do not significantly deviate from the actuarial tables which the policy premiums are based. Of course, there may be some exceptions, benefits and other matters we did not address but this is a simple way of discriminating between the two forms of life insurance and helps one understand how life insurance works and the potential profits available to insurers.

If you are older, male, obese, have lots of medical problems, smoke and live a risky lifestyle such as racing cars, you are much more likely to die sooner than a physically active younger, female with no medical problems, who has many family members living in good health into their 90's and 100's who are physically active and in good health. It does not guarantee that a younger female counterpart will live to an older age than her male counterpart, but based on historical and actuarial data, statistically the younger, healthier female will live longer and thus would pay life insurance premiums to the insurer for a longer period. Hence, the longer a person is likely to live, the more premiums that person will pay for the policy. This helps to explain why the premium rates can be lower for females for the same policy limits; they will likely make more payments because they live longer and are less risky from an insurer's standpoint. In addition, the insurer can invest the premium money longer and likely make more money from the "free use" of the money until the benefit must be paid out.

The opposite is true. Assume someone is 52 year-old male with severe heart disease that is in and out of hospitals frequently because of his heart condition, has high cholesterol, is very sedentary, continues to smoke and his parents both died in their 40's from heart disease along with many other relatives who died in their 20's, 30's, 40's and 50's. How long do you think this person is likely to live? Not very long based on statistics. While miracles happen and this person could live until he is 90, it is very unlikely. This person is unlikely to live much longer and hence would not pay premiums very long before he dies. Insurers would have to charge him an incredibly high rate to justify the risk. In fact, insurers may simply refuse to cover such a high-risk individual or only provide minimal amounts of coverage. This way of looking at human beings may sound mean, cruel or morbid, but this is how it is done. Life insurers look at people statistically and base their projections, pricing, policies etc. based on actuarial tables that are based on historical data and factors that influence life expectancies. In fairness, if life insurers ignored statistics and data, they would likely make bad business decisions, lose money and eventually go out of business. Another option would be for insurers to charge even more because they would want to guarantee a profit. Insurers want to assure that they will make enough money to cover all expenses and make enough profits to satisfy shareholders.

If health insurance companies are required to provide both health and life insurance, they would have a significant financial interest in keeping the insured person healthier and alive longer

Insurance companies have gotten pretty good at predicting life expectancies of people when they have accurate data and no "unexpected surprises" happen. You may say, unexpected things do happen and that is the reason people buy life insurance. In case a young parent or partner dies in a car accident or freak accident, the surviving spouse or young children will have the financial means to maintain their lifestyle and survive. This type of "unexpected" thing is taken into consideration in actuarial tables and formulas used by life insurers particularly when looking at companies that cover a statistically significant number of lives. An example of a surprise would be what happened in the 1980's with HIV/AIDS.

Up until the outbreak of HIV/AIDS, the chances of a young, otherwise healthy appearing, often active young man or woman with no known medical problems dying was very low. When the outbreak occurred and suddenly there were thousands of young people dying from an incurable disease, especially high in certain areas such as LA and NY, insurance companies lost a lot of money on these policies. Why? It was because the insurers had offered life insurance as they typically do. They based their premiums on the insured risks and life expectancy projections. So, when people expected to live into their 70's and 80's are dying in their 20's and 30's, the insurers must pay out large amounts of money 40, 50, or 60 years sooner than they projected. The insurer expected to collect much more money, and more importantly, expected to be able to use that money to invest and enjoy nice compounded returns over decades that would allow them to make up the difference between what they would have to pay out at time of death and what was collected, and make a nice profit. HIV/AIDS changed this.

Unlike the unexpected surprises that are considered in actuarial tables, HIV/AIDS was an unknown risk when the policies were written and agreed to contractually. The illness was not factored into the earlier actuarial tables and formulas. Add to this, HIV/AIDS did not just affect one or only a few insured, it affected thousands of people. Add to this, the disease affected more people in certain areas of the country. The insurers who offered life insurance in these areas were more affected than other companies that might not have had insured people in the areas most affected by this terrible virus and disease.

Even if the insurance company puts profits as their top priority and did not care about the patient, this hybrid model would incentivize better health and long-life that benefits everyone

As discussed earlier, there is a lot of "power in time" when it comes to investing. The longer the insured pays in premiums and the more time the insurance companies must invest the collected premiums before paying out policy benefits, the more money the life insurance companies tend to make. Here lies the strength of the hybrid insurance model. If we require health insurance to also cover the insured's life, then the insurance company that provides both health and life insurance has a significant financial interest in keeping the insured person healthier and alive longer. If the insurer does not provide quality healthcare and the insured gets sick and dies prematurely, the insurer stands to lose a lot of money. The insurer would only collect a fraction of what it expects to collect, would be able to invest for only a fraction of the time anticipated and the insurer would have to pay out the full amount of the life insurance policy sooner than expected. This is a double whammy and a big incentive to the insurer to make sure they do their best to keep the insured healthy and alive longer.

A hybrid lifetime health insurance-life insurance policy would provide lifetime coverage, avoid surprise price increases and give insurers a big financial incentive to keep you healthy and alive for a long time

By requiring insurers to provide both health and life insurance, you help align the insurer's best interest with the insured's best interest of good health and long life. One would hope that anyone, including insurers, would do what is best for patients. We also must be realistic and understand that different people and insurers might have different priorities. Even if one assumes that the insurance company puts profits as their top priority and doesn't care about the patient, this hybrid model will help create a situation where long-life and great healthcare benefits everyone including the insured, the public, society and the insurer. The insurer will maximize profits by keeping people healthy and alive for longer periods of time.

Our current broken healthcare and health insurance structure does not provide people with long-term security. Insurers can choose to not renew your policy, can require you to get the insurers' approval for evaluation, testing and treatment, can increase your rates by amounts that you may not know until soon before it goes into effect and typically only guarantees coverage for a one year period at a time. This system is not optimal. In fact, it is failing the people it should be helping: the insured public. We could force a bunch of government price controls but often government is not the best when it comes to doing what is most innovative or effective. Government is often very inefficient and ineffective. However, government can help create policy that creates an environment that encourages competition, innovation and creative thought and allows smart, resourceful and hard-working people to figure out solutions better than we might imagine. Certainly, the bar is currently so low, it should not be too difficult to improve.

The long-term policy period model was introduced, and we focused mostly on the lifetime policy model. The lifetime insurance model would solve the issue of denial of renewal by the insurer and guarantee healthcare coverage so long as the policy premiums are paid. It would also prevent the insured, public, from surprise price increases of policy premiums and provide predictability so families can accurately make spending budgets. The potential drawback, "sinister" possibility of the long-term policy, was that it may sometimes be in the best financial interest of the insurer for the high user of healthcare patient, or insured, to die. If the insured died, the insurer would no longer have to pay for any health care costs. Of course, one would hope insurers would not put profits ahead of life and good health, but we must consider as many possibilities as possible, no matter how likely or unlikely. One solution might be to shorten the policy period which would lessen the cost obligation to insurers when compared to a lifetime policy. The insurer would only have to provide coverage for the remaining time on the health insurance policy and then could be free from the financial liability. This may help with the concern of insurer benefiting from insured dying but only a little. It would also create a whole new problem. It would introduce one of the biggest drawbacks of our current system into the lifetime model. If insurers only committed to a 10-year term, then if the patient contracted a chronic illness that had high costs associated with care, the insurer would be responsible but only for the remainder of the policy period. Then what? The insurer would charge a higher premium, not renew or try to get out of the policy as early as legally possible. If this happens, it is likely the insured would have difficulty finding insurance from another insurance company. If they did, the person would likely have a huge increase in policy premium compared to before because their risk profile is now much worse than it was when they signed up for their first 10-year policy before contracting the costly chronic condition. Therefore, the lifetime policy period seems optimal if we want to maximize population health. It is most likely to be the optimal time period that would prevent surprise price increases. Another and probably more effective way to put people at ease, that insurers would not benefit by the insured dying as opposed to living, is making insurers provide life insurance. This combination of a lifetime health insurance policy with upfront rates from year 1 to year 100 combined with a life insurance policy of a significant amount would make the most sense and provide the most security to the public. A hybrid lifetime health insurance-life insurance policy would provide lifetime coverage, avoid surprise price increases and give insurers a big financial incentive to keep you healthy and alive for a long time.

There are many other factors that could be included. There could be buyout clauses, mechanisms or certain factors that could allow insurers to renegotiate terms, including compensations if changes are made as value of original contract would change with contract changes, secondary markets, what happens if insurers are sold or merge, financial and other incentives to people for staying healthy. These factors were intentionally not discussed in this book but worth mentioning as there are so many possibilities and options to improve our healthcare system.

Chapter 4 Talking Points:

- Increased competition of insurance companies is good for the public and all qualified insurers should be allowed to sell insurance across state lines and across the country.
- Insurance is intended to spread out financial risk of the insured individual, thus providing security and value to the public.
- By shifting more and more of the risks back to the insured via deductibles, co-payments, co-insurance, higher costs if a patient chooses an out-of-network physician, insurers are acting contrary to the fundamental reason insurance exists.
- Lifetime health insurance policies with upfront pricing allow the public to have lifelong security and predictability that is desired but not currently available
- Whole life insurance is more expensive than term life insurance.
- A person may be much better off financially buying term life insurance, as opposed to whole life insurance, and investing the cost savings in an Standards and Poor (S&P) index fund.
- Hybrid Lifetime Health and Life Insurance will incentivize insurance companies to cover all necessary testing and treatment and keep people healthier and alive longer.
- Hybrid Health & Life Insurance could cause significant financial disincentives if a patient is unhealthy and dies prematurely.

Chapter Five:
DIRECT & EMPLOYER CARE ORGANIZATIONS...
AN INSURANCE ALTERNATIVE

The Direct Care Organization (DCO) model is based on a community, group of individuals or group of businesses taking charge and arranging for or directly providing any healthcare that is needed by its members. It is intended to be owned or operated by whoever is currently paying for healthcare. It can be owned by a community, by the residents of the community who pay for healthcare themselves, employers, employees of a company, physicians, hospitals or a combination of any of these. Regardless of ownership, the idea is that whatever a member (employee or person who pays a membership fee to be part of the DCO) or patient needs, it is provided directly to the patient without unnecessary delays or need for approvals, unnecessary paperwork, waits or additional costs to the patient i.e. significantly reducing or elimination of co-pays, co-insurance, deductibles, etc. There are no insurance premiums but instead, in order to receive care at a DCO, one needs to be a member and membership can be paid by an individual, by an employer or by anyone else on a member's behalf.

To maximize the potential savings, the DCO is owned and operated by the people whom it is meant to serve thus eliminating as many "middlemen" as possible. It just seems to make sense and would be easier for employers, who fund most of the premiums of private healthcare policies, to own or run healthcare programs independently or in conjunction with other employers or payers of healthcare services. Of course, it can also be done in conjunction with physicians, hospitals or others in healthcare, but this is not recommended.

DCOs are different. They are designed to remove as many of the inefficiencies and processes that add little to no value in healthcare and do not tolerate the waste, high costs, inefficiencies and lack of services of hospitals, urgent cares, clinics, physician offices or the current healthcare complex. Think of it as a place where a patient can get quality care, with minimal to no wait for any service, ability to get whatever test, lab or imaging with no question or additional cost and convenient 24/7 service. Think of it being a place that is built for you, caters to you and answers to you because it is often owned by you. It is a way of delivering care and service that is member obsessed© and different from what any hospital, insurer or other for-profit or governmental entity offers.

A DCO is patient obsessed© and flexible. It does whatever is best and most convenient for the patients and members

Employer, or employee, owned DCOs would be known as Employer Care Organizations (ECOs) or Employee Care Organization (ECO), and one could refer to it as an "ECO system" i.e. an employee would get the tests and care they need in the ecosystem (ECO system). An ECO is one type of a DCO but work essentially the same. It can be owned by a single company, a co-op of companies or by the employees that pay into it. There are many ways to structure it. It is a new, better way of doing things. It puts the employee patients' health and best interest above all else. It is "employee-obsessed©." It helps align everyone to benefit from the same thing; making healthcare simple, the best it can be for the patient or employee and the best value. The DCO model makes it easier for employees to access care, shortens waiting times and removes unnecessary steps that do not add value to the patient or the employee's care.

Another way of looking at the mission of a DCO is to think of how to do the right thing for the employee (patient) or make things as you would want them to be or done if the patient was your mother, your child or any loved one. The primary mission and purpose of a DCO is to maximize the health and well-being of its members, not maximize profits of the DCO. As you may recall, in 2018, the average cost of healthcare per employee with a family plan was about $20,000. If a company employees 1000 people, that employer and its employees are spending $20,000,000 per year on healthcare. If the employer employs 2,000, then $40,000,000 per year. It doesn't take long to realize how much money is involved in healthcare. Many businesses understand costs and the importance of cost containment and efficient usage and optimization. Why not apply these same skills in the healthcare world? Add to that, if businesses joined and formed partnerships and co-operatives, many of the costs could be shared and reduced on a per employee basis.

Even small and medium sized employers can participate and benefit along with their employees. If smaller employers cooperate and band together in the same geographic area, the businesses could pool resources and develop a direct care organization that could provide all sorts of health services, laboratory services, imaging and treatments in a more effective and efficient manner than their employees currently receive. For example, if businesses that employed 5,000 in an area pooled their resources and created a "direct care co-op (DCC)," they would have $100,000,000 to use to provide the healthcare that is needed for those 5,000 employees. The DCO could build a fully functioning micro hospital, hire their own physicians and other providers, hire therapists and dieticians, buy their own laboratory, X-ray, imaging and diagnostic equipment including ultrasound, computerized tomography (CT), magnetic resonance imaging (MRI), positron emission tomography (PET), catheterization labs, surgical centers, etc. For efficiency, the physical location would be centrally located and house all physician and non-physician providers' offices and imaging, laboratory services. In addition, the DCO would offer 24/7 access and care to all employees via Telehealth, or in-person, and allow after hours imaging, testing and other services as need and

appropriateness arises. The idea is that the DCO is patient obsessed©
and flexible and does whatever is best and most convenient for the
patients and members.

The DCO can provide just about any medical and healthcare service that
any employee may need including education and active management
and incentives that promote healthier diets, a healthier lifestyle and
improved health. Here's the exciting part... if managed properly, the
employees of these employers would immediately experience better
care, more convenience, less hassles, little to any denials, low to no co-
pays or deductibles and would save money. Sound too good to be true?
It gets better. After the first year or two, care will remain constant or
improve but costs will go down substantially because the start-up costs
have been paid off or paid down substantially. The efficiencies built into
this model are predicted to save 10-40% of what is currently being spent
on healthcare and provide equivalent, or superior healthcare, to what is
currently being delivered.

For illustration purposes, we will make up a possible scenario for how
things might work in the traditional insurance and healthcare model;
the current broken healthcare system we have. Let's say Mary works for
Company A and has lots of headaches. She has not seen a doctor in over
a year. Mary calls the PCP's office and cannot be seen for two weeks.
Two weeks later, Mary takes off work and goes to see her primary care
physician (PCP) who attempts to treat her. Unfortunately, her
headaches continue and become more frequent and remain severe. She
sees her PCP again. Mary's PCP recommends that Mary obtain a CT scan
of the brain and see a neurologist, a specialist that treats migraines and
other disorders involving the nervous system. Mary tries to schedule a
CT scan and an appointment but discovers that the imaging center
charges $1,200 for the brain CT scan. She informs the imaging center
that she has insurance with Insurer A. The imaging center states they
will try to get authorization from Insurer A so Mary can get the scan and
the costs be covered by Insurer A. Mary must wait to hear back before
she gets her brain CT. This authorization may be given or refused by

Insurer A. Insurer A may require more reasoning or justification for the brain CT. If the Insurer approves, then the CT can be scheduled, and Mary can come in when the imaging center schedules her to have the scan. This may take a day or two or it could take a week or more. Assume it is approved and scheduled, Mary takes off work and comes in for her scan. In the meanwhile, she has called for an appointment with the neurologist that her PCP recommended. Unfortunately, that neurologist does not accept Mary's insurance. Apparently, Mary's insurance company was willing to only pay 1/3 of what the neurologist typically charges for his services, so the neurologist refused to accept Mary's insurance company's lower rate. Mary has the option of paying the full fee of the neurologist out of pocket and possibly not even have that count towards her deductible. Mary has the option of seeing a different neurologist or Mary may choose to try to put up with the pain. Mary calls Insurer A and tries to see if there is some way, she can see the specialist that her PCP recommended. She trusts her PCP's opinion and wants to see the neurologist her PCP recommended. After calling Insurer A, waiting on hold, verifying her information, explaining her situation speaking to the representative, she is told Insurer will not pay for Mary to see that neurologist. Frustrated, Mary thanks the representative and cannot understand why she pays over $400 a month, in addition to what her employer pays, for health insurance and cannot see a specialist that her PCP, who has examined her twice for these symptoms, recommended. Mary asked for and was given the name of a neurologist that Insurer A will cover, we will call her Neurologist B. The next day, Mary calls Neurologist B's office to make an appointment. She is told she needs a referral so hangs up and calls her PCP's office and informs them. The PCP's office staff informs her they will make a referral and in fact even offer to call the neurologist's office for Mary. Mary is told that Neurologist B's office will call her with the appointment time. A couple days later while at work, Mary gets a voice message from Neurologist B's office. At lunch, Mary decides to call to make the appointment as her headache continue to be bad. She reaches Neurologist B's office and finds out that the earliest she can be seen is 8 weeks. Mary explains how much pain she is in and what she has already gone through and is told they may be able to fit her in in 4 weeks. Mary waits 4 weeks, still with pain off and on before she can see neurologist B. Mary must take off work go see her PCP 2 times during the wait. Mary even made one emergency room visit because she was in so much pain and it was after hours. During that visit, she had an emergency CT scan, bloodwork and received IV medications to treat her pain. She called her PCP and the answering service informed Mary that she should go to the ER if she felt it was an emergency.

A month after her call with the Neurologist's office, Mary takes a sick day in order to see Neurologist B. After being examined and her CT scan of the brain that was done during her ER visit reviewed, the neurologist prescribed a different medication for her headaches and ordered an MRI scan of the brain. Mary mentioned what happened with the CT requiring authorization so the neurologist reassures her that her office will call the insurer and get authorization. She was told to return for a follow up visit after she had her MRI scan. Mary does not hear anything for about a week but then hears from Neurologist B's office. Insurer A has denied authorization for the MRI. Mary calls Insurer A to see if she can get approval but is told it is not indicated. She goes around and around with the representative and even asks to speak to a supervisor to see if that will help. She is told a supervisor will call her back. Frustrated, Mary calls the imaging center to ask how much the MRI as ordered will cost and gives the name of her insurer. She is told the MRI is $3,000. Mary realizes she cannot afford that much and waits to hear from the Insurer A. A few days later the supervisor calls and after verifying her information again, telling her story, explaining her pain and the hassles she has been through and pleading her case, the supervisor states she will need more information from the ordering neurologist. Mary calls Neurologist B and explains what has happened and that Insurer A needs information and provides the office with the supervisor's name and contact info. In a few days, Mary calls Insurer A to check on the status of the MRI that the Neurologist B had ordered and after verifying her information, explaining why she was calling and spending about an hour on the phone, Mary was happy to discover the

MRI would be approved. She thanked the representative and called the imaging center and scheduled the appointment for the MRI scan. Once again, Mary had to provide her information, insurance information and was given an appointment 3 days later. Three days later, Mary took off work and had her MRI scan and called Neurologist B to schedule her follow up appointment as she was instructed during her first visit with the neurologist. Neurologist B's office scheduled her 2 weeks later. Fortunately, Mary was feeling better. The new medication that the neurologist had prescribed seemed to be helping. Two weeks later, Mary saw Neurologist B for follow up and was feeling much better. The frequency and severity of the headaches were much better and tolerable. Neurologist B went over the MRI findings. Fortunately, everything appeared to be OK. The neurologist was pleased that she was able to rule out more serious causes of the headaches that Mary had described. Mary was told to make a follow up appointment in 6 months but to call before if she had any problems.

Thankfully, Mary's symptoms improved, and her tests did not show anything more serious. That's the good news. Here's the unfortunate part of the story. Mary, in her time of need, had to hassle with making numerous calls, for appointments, authorizations and discussions to try to get what her attending physicians, who examined her, had recommended. She had to fight with the insurance company to allow her to get what the experts told her she needed. She had to wait for appointments, referrals, imaging and ultimately getting the medications that would help her condition. In addition, no telling how much she had to pay for co-pays, co-insurance and in deductibles. It is reported that the average deductible in the US in 2018 amongst all workers with employer-sponsored insurance plans was $1,350,[41] but many other plans have deductibles of $5,000, $7,000, $10,000 or more. According to information provided during the ACEP LAC Conference in Washington, DC in May 2019, a typical deductible is $7,000. Applying this deductible to Mary, she likely had to pay the full amount of the costs of her care from the PCP, neurologist, CT, MRI and medications. This could be as high as $5,000 or more for the care, doctors' appointments, ER visit, imaging and medication, even though she has insurance. This does not include the 5-7 days she had to miss work to attend doctors' appointments or to get the imaging performed that was ordered. Fortunately for Mary, her MRI did not show anything bad or that required surgery or aggressive treatment, but what if it had? This would have been unfortunate. Added to this, the treatment that may have been needed would have been delayed by the delayed diagnosis caused by the inefficiencies inherent to the current insurance industry and broken healthcare system that made Mary wait to get the tests that her doctors ordered.

An Employer Care Organization takes out waste and inefficiencies that are inherent to our traditional insurance models

Now let's imagine if Mary was a member of a DCO and see how Mary's experience might have been different. Mary would still have a deduction from her check for her membership in the DCO as with her current insurance plan. When Mary developed a headache and wanted to be seen by a PCP, she has the option of scheduling an appointment to be seen in the office or being seen immediately within minutes by a PCP via Telehealth that is provided by her DCO. She could do so from home or during her lunch break at work so she would not have to miss work. In fact, she could be seen 24/7/365.

Should she make an appointment to be seen in person, she would be seen within 24-48 hours, typically the same day, as the physicians are paid for this very reason, to be available specifically for employees of the companies who make up the DCO. If done via telephone, online or via mobile device app, Mary would be seen within minutes. When she was seen, whether in person or via Telehealth, if the PCP felt she needed to have a CT scan and be evaluated by a neurologist as was case in previous example, the appointment and CT would be scheduled then with no need for authorization; the DCO assures that any referrals and testing ordered by the physicians of the DCO will be covered with no need for further authorization if done at the DCO. If Mary was seen in person by the PCP located within the DCO complex, she could have the CT scan performed immediately after leaving the PCP's office as no authorization is needed with the DCO. Mary could literally walk from her PCP's office to the imaging center located within the same medical complex and have her CT the same day, often within minutes. If seen by a Telehealth physician and the doctor felt Mary needed a CT scan, Mary could have gone to have the CT scan at any time that was convenient for her 24 hours a day. At Mary's convenience, she could have gone to the DCO's imaging center after work to have the necessary scan without having to get approvals, calling to schedule or jumping through unnecessary "hoops." If the DCO's physician orders it, it needs no further approval.

With the DCO, Mary would be scheduled to be seen by the specialist, in this case the neurologist, within 48 hours or sooner if necessary. Mary even has the option of being evaluated by the neurologist via Telehealth if she prefers or if it is more convenient to her. Should Mary decide to go to the neurologist's office or has not already had the CT recommended by the PCP, she could have the CT scheduled to be done an hour or two before her neurologist's visit, since imaging is located within the DCO complex where the neurologist is located. Whatever is more convenient to or best for Mary is what the DCO would do.

Once seen by the neurologist and the specialist determines Mary needs an MRI scan, as was the case described in the example of how things work today, she goes directly to the imaging area of the DCO complex and gets it. No authorization needed, no phone calls and long waits, no discussion with insurance reps, no wait for scheduling, no need to take another day off work to come in, no hassles. After the scan is done, the scan and/or MRI report can be sent to, or accessed by the neurologist. If early enough, necessary and Mary wishes, she can even wait for the scan to be read by a radiologist and then walk the report back to the neurologist to get follow up and closure the same day to get answers and to avoid having to wait or returning on another day and missing work.

The good news is Mary starts to feel better. Her headache is starting to get better, she is re-assured everything has checked out well and she is thankful she was able to get seen so quickly and not having to go through all of the hassles that she has heard friends, who have "good" traditional insurance, have gone through to try and get necessary healthcare. She is thankful she only missed 1-2 days of work instead of the 5-7 she might have had she had traditional health insurance. Finally, she is thankful because the cost of seeing her PCP, a specialist and getting a CT and an MRI was less than $500 to her.

With the DCO model, Mary has seen a PCP and a specialist within 2-4 days or less and obtained a CT and MRI scan as opposed to the 1-2-month ordeal she might experience with traditional health insurance. With the DCO model, Mary missed 5 days less of work and she had to pay about 10% of what she might have had to pay with traditional insurance model. Mary is much better off being a member of her employer's ECO system than having traditional insurance.

The employer is much better off with the ECO model. For no extra cost, the ECO model allows Mary to get the same, and one could argue even better care and service as she would with the traditional insurance model, without having to miss so much work. That is 5 extra days of work production from Mary with the ECO model as compared to the traditional insurance model. Mary feels better sooner, which is a good thing. First, it makes sense that an employee who feels good is more likely to do his/her job better than if they are at work feeling sick or with a bad headache. Second, employer wants their employee to be happy. Happy employees are more likely to be productive employees. They perform better and are more likely to be loyal to the company. Happy employees have less reason to change jobs which saves businesses money in training and lower productivity.

It is estimated that the ECO model, if done properly, could ultimately save 10-40% annually in healthcare costs

Sounds almost too good to be true. How can this work? The simplest way to answer this is that the Employer Care Organization takes out a lot of the waste and inefficiencies that are inherent to our current traditional insurance model. It is patient obsessed©. It aligns the interests for what is best for patients (employees) and those who are the gatekeepers of healthcare. Currently, employers and employees pay a lot of money for employees to have health insurance, yet the current insurance model, either by design, poor management skills, the insurers' attempt to maximize profits, or other unexplained reasons, seems to put up barriers for patients to access care. The insured often must jump through many hoops, make appointments, be inconvenienced, seek prior insurance authorization, and argue with insurance company representatives to get what a treating physician, who has examined them, has ordered and often pay ridiculously large sums of money in addition to what they already pay in insurance premiums.

If one keeps it simple and understands how the current insurance model works, it makes it easy to understand. Once insurance companies collect premiums and have a big pile of money, the less money the insurance companies must give to others, the more of that pile of money the insurance companies get to keep. The insurance companies use some of that money for marketing efforts, paying employee salaries, to pay the CEOs and other leaders who sometimes make hundreds of millions of dollars. Any money they have to pay for an insured patient to see a doctor, have a blood test, have an X-ray, CT, MRI, mammogram, PAP smear, surgery, joint replacement, brace, walker or any other healthcare expense, is less potential profits for insurers. Insurance companies are likely owned by shareholders and they want to make money on their investment. In the eyes of shareholders, healthcare is not a charity, it is big business and they want to make "big" money; the more the better.

In the DCO model, your membership dues help pay for the doctors' pay, the equipment, the micro-hospital, the imaging center, therapists, dieticians, laboratory etc. Many of the costs that don't add any value to the healthcare of the patient are removed such as people who review and deny authorization for referrals, imaging, testing, etc. The administrative costs of the insurance company are removed because there is none. The profits of the insurance company are removed. The costs and profits of many other parts of the health ecosystem are reduced or eliminated and used for your care and convenience. So, all the waste and profits of the traditional imaging center, laboratory testing, coding and billing personnel at the insurer, doctors' offices, imaging centers and labs are drastically reduced or eliminated and can be used for better care and service to the DCO members.

In the first year or two, the DCO uses the collected monthly payments that ordinarily would go to insurance premiums, to pay for most, if not all, of the costs including building the micro-hospital and buying expensive equipment while still providing treatment to those who require it. Once paid for, the hospital and start up equipment don't have to be bought every year. This frees up money to lowering premiums, acquiring more equipment or providing more services. Based on Kaiser Family Foundation (KFF) statistics, premiums for traditional employer sponsored health plans have increased 78% from 2000-2006, 37% from 2006-2012 and 25% from 2012-2018.[42] That's 233% of the amount paid in 2000. Even if health premiums continue their current pace, we will continue to spend more and more each year at a much faster rate than wages so patients will have an even more difficult time paying their portion of premiums, deductibles, co-pays and co-insurance. People will have less money for food, housing and other necessities. With the DCO model, these excessive premium increases can be eliminated, and premiums could go down along with co-pays, co-insurance and deductibles; that is something unheard of in health insurance in our current system.

Another advantage is that the ECO can help return money to the participating company or employees. In the traditional insurance model, if there is excess money left over at the end of the year, this might be used as a dividend payments to the insurers' shareholders, be used to pay bonuses to CEOs or other executives, for a stock buy-back or acquisitions. In the ECO model, it could be used to buy additional equipment or expand services that would benefit employees. Another option for the ECO is to return money to the employers or employees who pay into the ECO. In the example of a ECO consisting of 5,000 employees paying $20,000 a year in healthcare expenses, that is an annual working budget of $100,000,000.00. It is estimated that the ECO model, if done properly, could ultimately save 10-40% annually in healthcare costs. If we assume a conservative savings of 20%, that is an annual savings of $20,000,000. That's a lot of money. Perhaps providing bonuses to employees for living healthier, using it as a slush fund for the employees' benefit such as a health savings account (HSA) or retirement fund, obtaining catastrophic policies for all of its members or simply keeping the money as a reserve for the ECO to offset any future unexpected costs. Another big benefit of the DCO is that the typical annual premium increases that occur with traditional insurance can be reduced or even eliminated. Even if there are increases in the cost of healthcare that cannot be controlled, the ECO is insulated to some degree because it owns components of healthcare which reduces some of the exposure that employees and employers are currently at risk with the traditional insurance model.

By using an ECO, people could get better care, faster care and save a lot of money

These are just some of the financial benefits of the DCO. Remember the care and convenience can be much better than the current traditional insurance model. One might argue the care and convenience of a DCO would justify a higher cost. With the DCO, you can get great care, great convenience, pay less and feel secure and cared for. Also, the DCO can be owned by the employer or employee so it can be adjusted to best serve the employee much easier than an insurance company would adjust it.

Some pushback to a DCO may be that it is unproven and will not work. Until we try, we will not know but intuitively, it makes sense. Even if it were done and was not done perfectly, say mediocre, it still would be much better than what we currently have with the traditional insurance model. There is so much waste, fluff and cushioning in premiums that pay for things that provide no benefit to the employer or employee. With the DCO, the money collected is used for the patient and for healthcare. The priority for everyone involved is to keep people healthy and if they get sick, to get them seen and treated faster and with better service and care.

Some might say that people can't expect deductibles to be eliminated without premiums going up 100% or more. They might argue that if insurers pay $1000 or $2,000 for a scan, you can't expect them to not deny the scan or allow it without making the patient pay a good portion of the total. This argument is almost laughable. This is part of the misinformation that benefits insurers. People may be afraid and feel they need insurance companies or that insurance companies protect them. This may be what the insurance companies have trained us to believe or the "Kool Aid" the insurers want us to drink.

Let's use an example of a CT scan to illustrate this point i.e. a CT of the abdomen and pelvis. The imaging center may charge $1,200 for this study. What you don't know is the insurer may negotiate a deal with the imaging center for $600 so long as the imaging center charges the patient a co-pay of $100. The co-pay serves two purposes for the insurer. One, it lessens what the insurer must pay. Two, it might discourage a patient from having the test. If the patient must pay $100, the patient might decide not to have the study. The patient may not have $100 to spend. If the patient doesn't have the scan, the insurer just saved $500. But what is the "real cost" of that CT scan? Forget the mark up and the built-in profit of the imaging center. Ignore the cost of the building, the license, the marketing and all the other costs for a minute. For a DCO that has already bought and paid for the CT scanner and the other items, what is the additional cost to the DCO to perform that one additional CT scan? In economics, this is known as the "variable costs" of that CT scan, as opposed to the total costs. Total costs include the variable costs and the fixed costs. The fixed costs are costs such as what the CT scanner and equipment cost to buy or lease, the service agreement for the scanner, the salaries of people already working, rent, etc. But since all the other fixed costs are incurred already, whether we do this additional CT scan or not, really it is the variable costs that I will discuss to make a point. Variable costs are only the additional costs incurred to do that additional one CT scan. The variable cost of that $1,200 CT is probably less than $20. So, in the traditional insurance model, when you pay your co-pay, you are paying about 5 times what that additional scan costs that imaging center to perform. This does not even include the $500 more the insurance company pays to the imaging center. So, in the traditional insurance model, $600 is spent on a $20 scan. In the DCO, $20 could be spent and the remaining $580 can be saved to be used for other healthcare. This gives you an idea of the potential impact and savings a DCO model can have to you, employers and society. $20 vs. $600, over 95% savings.

Right off the top, at least 20% of the money spent by employers for healthcare does not go to care at all. 20% goes to non-healthcare expenses

Keep in mind, we used a conservative figure for the imaging center's typical charge in our example; it is commonly much higher than $1,200. In fairness, the fixed costs must be covered for the model to be sustainable over time. Even if we quadruple the variable costs for fixed costs, the cost of the CT scan would be about $100, still only a fraction of what is currently being paid for the study. If we go crazy and build in a cushion of 1000% of the variable cost used in this example, that would place the total cost to the DCO of the CT scan of about $220, still less than half what the current discounted cost is in the example used for our current broken healthcare system. It is less than 20% of the $1,200 non-discounted charge. Unlike the current healthcare complex, the goal of an ECO is not to maximize profits. The goal of the ECO is to maximize employees' health, prevent illness and maximize savings through smart, innovative and efficient care.

Another potential criticism of the DCO model might be, what happens if someone has a very expensive illness or condition such as cancer, require an organ transplant, etc. Such conditions can cost well into the hundreds of thousands of dollars. This is a valid point and should be addressed. The simple answer is the DCO would have a built-in catastrophic policy that covers patients for anyone who uses over $100,000 each year. Such patients could receive the necessary care from a facility able to treat whatever the patient needed or beyond the capability of the DCO. To use an insurance term, the actuarial tables and data show that such occurrences occur but are very unusual. The actual cost to care for most people's healthcare is much lower than what they pay in premiums. Remember, insurance is to spread risk. If 1 in 1,000,000 get a rare and expensive to treat disease, it is very unlikely you will get that disease i.e. you will be the one. But someone will and if they do not have insurance or some other protection, they will be most likely be financially wiped out and unable to afford treatment. A DCO can take care of most anything but perhaps not everything. For such rare, unusual and expensive diseases, illnesses or injuries, the DCO would obtain catastrophic coverage from a liability carrier to cover any illness, injury or disease for any costs that exceed $100,000. Because almost all healthcare will be far less than $100,000 in any given year, insurers can offer such coverage for a very small fraction of the costs of health insurance with deductibles of $7000 or even $20,000. Of course, the DCO would cover the deductible or first $20,000 or $100,000 of costs before the catastrophic policy kicked in. The DCO will obtain this on behalf of all its members. Thus, if any member of the DCO requires any healthcare, the DCO can provide it. If the costs exceed $100,000 which would likely financially devastate the DCO employee member and could potentially financially hurt the DCO, the ECO and employee member will be protected by the catastrophic policy. If the DCO is large enough and has enough members, it could justify assuming this risk as current large insurance companies do. In my example of 5,000 employees that generates $100,000,000 in membership or subscription fees, it would be unlikely for a member to have a catastrophic condition that occurs 1 in a million. But just in case, the catastrophic policy is there. Of course, various DCOs throughout the country could form a co-op or pool their members and resources to create their own catastrophe fund to cover any member of any of the participating DCOs who develops any catastrophic illness or injury.

One might notice that the DCO is not referred to as insurance and the monthly amounts to be a member of the DCO (or ECO) or pay for the DCO are not referred to as premiums. This is intentional. Insurance is a specifically defined thing with potential legal ramifications. There are terms and laws specific to insurance. Not just anyone can sell insurance; the insurance industry is heavily regulated, and trade is restricted to a certain degree. Restriction of trade can hurt the public. A DCO is not an insurance company. DCOs can eliminate the need for traditional insurance and offer services that are superior to what an insurance company can offer for similar or even higher costs. A person can decide to choose the DCO route, and become a member and pay membership dues, or traditional health insurance with a health insurance company and pay insurance premiums. Choice is good. After weighing the benefits, costs and drawbacks to each, it is believed many will realize that joining a DCO is the best choice for them and their families. Legislators need to assure that DCOs can exist and offer consumers more choices.

Another advantage of an ECO being self-funded by the employer and employee is that it avoids some of the problems inherent to the current traditional insurance model. For example, insurance company interactions with people, physicians, hospitals etc., are all too often centered on payment issues. Is this covered? Will the insurer pay for that? Whether for a test, referral, scan or telehealth visit. With the DCO, the focus is more on patient health and what is easiest and best for the person. Remember, a DCO, or ECO system is all about the patient, it is patient-obsessed©. What will help employees be seen sooner? What will help patients feel better faster? What will make things easiest or most convenient to the patient? What can we do to keep members of the DCO healthy? The DCO model is not just a different model; it is a different way of thinking and providing healthcare. The DCO model simplifies things and most importantly, it improves healthcare and makes employee members, employers, providers, and society better off.

Large employers can become more involved in healthcare. Whether as an "insurance company," as a DCO or otherwise. Laws and regulators may not allow employers to become insurers for various reason but maybe government and society need to re-evaluate this and determine what is best for the public given the state-of-affairs in healthcare today. A DCO model, membership or subscription model that allows members or participants to receive care "free" or for minimal to no cost at the time of need so long as they have paid their membership fees. By pre-paying, many unnecessary costs that are inherent to our current broken healthcare system can be eliminated. DCOs would in a sense compete with insurers but in a different way. Insurers compete to try to maximize profits as a primary role. DCOs compete to maximize health as its primary role and may sacrifice profits in order to achieve its goal.

Employers are already involved with and paying for healthcare as 152 million non-elderly people get their insurance through employer-sponsored insurance.[43] Employers often pay for at least part of the premiums to obtain insurance for their employees. Employers are already paying the insurance company for health insurance coverage. Healthcare costs are going up at a rate faster than wages, revenues and most every other thing; it is becoming a bigger and bigger part of expenses for employers. At the current pace, healthcare costs could financially ruin companies and cause them to fail. Given it is becoming a bigger and bigger expense and could potentially jeopardize the viability of a business, businesses now have more and more incentives and reasons to get more involved and try to save money. An ECO is a great option that every employer needs to consider.

Unlike the current healthcare complex, the goal of an ECO is not to maximize profits, but to maximize employees' health, prevent illness and maximize savings through innovative and efficient care

Insurance companies do not provide care. They are a middleman. They sell policies, collect premiums, and then contract with others to provide services to the people that they sold policies to, the insured. What makes them so good? One could argue they are not good at all. They are quite inefficient. It is estimated that insurance companies spend about 20% on administrative costs, overhead and profits. So right off the top, 20% of the money spent by employers for healthcare does not go to care at all. 20% goes to non-healthcare expenses. This does not even consider the enormous amount spent on other non-healthcare items listed as "quality improvements" that can be open to interpretation. Nor does not take into consideration all the "costs" of healthcare i.e. the large sums that many other healthcare complex players take out for over-priced services and profits.

Chapter 5 Talking Points:

- Direct Care Organizations (DCO) are a new way of providing healthcare to employees or members at a lower cost and in a more convenient patient-obsessed© manner. Unlike insurance, they are primarily concerned with maximizing your health not maximizing profits.
- Employer or Employee Care Organizations (ECO) or "ECO system," a form of DCOs, do not require authorizations, do not deny testing or do not deny imaging. If your ECO physician orders it, you get it. Care is available 24/7 in person or via telehealth anytime-anywhere.
- Healthcare costs have increased each year and outpaced inflation and wages. DCOs can not only slow rate increases, but also can cause absolute costs to decrease.
- DCOs eliminate many of the inefficiencies and waste associated with health insurance and healthcare.
- DCOs reduce, or eliminate, deductibles, co-payments, co-insurance and other additional charges and fees. They can potentially save employers or employees 20-40% in healthcare costs.

Chapter Six:
PHYSICIAN AND NON-PHYSICIAN PROVIDERS

Physician are a very important component of healthcare. Not only are they the ones who have the sacred doctor-patient relationship with their patients, examine patients and offer treatment, but also, they are often the people who determine what labs, images, tests, surgeries or other expensive diagnostic or treatments patients may need. It has been said that the most expensive and costly item in healthcare is the pen. This is a reference to the pen that a physician uses to order labs, imaging, treatments or other studies that can. While physicians and other non-physician providers are paid and are part of the costs of healthcare, this is only a small part of the costs, reported to be 20% or less of the healthcare dollar.[44] The vast majority of healthcare expenses are not paid to doctors and other NPPs, but occur as a result of a doctor or other NPP's order for a test, referral to a specialist or facility, determination that a procedure is needed or recommendation, or ordering of various treatments. Perhaps with the advancements of technology, it could be said that the most-costly thing today in medicine is a mouse, tablet, voice recognition device or other tool used to order tests and treatments for patients by their treating physician or non-physician providers.

I have already pointed out that the term "provider" or "healthcare provider" is often used by many payers to include any person or entity that provides any healthcare treatment or services i.e. physicians, nurse practitioners, physician assistants, hospitals, imaging centers, laboratories, physical therapists and centers, treatment centers, etc. Insurers, government and even some physicians, nurse practitioners and physician assistants use this term. I believe this is confusing, especially to the public and should be avoided. Most would agree there is a significant difference between physicians and non-physicians in terms of the length of their training, the amount and depth of information and subject matter, the particular specialty related information taught and the knowledge base that is expected, the qualifications, degrees and certifications of the faculty that teaches, trains and oversees them, etc. Nurse practitioners and physician assistants have been called "midlevels," "advanced practice practitioners (APPs)" and "extenders" to differentiate them from physicians (medical doctors-MDs and doctors of osteopathy-DOs).

Some nurse practitioners and physician assistants have pushed to eliminate these terms as some find them to be inappropriate, insulting or demeaning. Others find the terms mid-levels, extenders and APP acceptable. In order to keep the peace and not offend those who may be offended, and for the purposes of this book, I will use the term non-physician healthcare provider or non-physician provider (NPP) to refer to nurse practitioners and physician assistants. Should I slip, the terms can be substituted for one another i.e. NPP, APP, mid-level, physician-extender. The term NPP will not ordinarily be used in this book to refer to hospitals, imaging centers, laboratories or other entities within healthcare that are referred to as "providers" by insurance policies, contract management groups or various contract used in healthcare.

The term physician refers to doctors of both medicine and osteopathy. The term physicians and doctors refer to the same people and can be used interchangeably; it seems to be more of a personal preference. I doubt that most physicians are offended to be called either. I hope this helps clarify any confusion that one might have regarding physicians or NPPs. Confusion is typically not good for patients or anyone in healthcare.

To illustrate just one of the many examples of how our current healthcare system is broken, an example of reimbursement for someone involved in a motor vehicle accident will be discussed. Often after motor vehicle accidents, the occupants of the accidents are brought to the emergency room by emergency medical services (EMS) immobilized in a cervical collar and on a hard backboard. This is done as a precaution in the event any spinal injury exists and to prevent further injury, possibly even paralysis from an unstable spinal fracture. Many emergency physicians have believed for years that patients are often unnecessarily placed in this very uncomfortable immobilization but that is for another discussion.

When a patient comes into the emergency room by ambulance with spinal immobilization precautions, it is very routine that these patients have X-ray imaging of their cervical (neck), thoracic (upper back) and lumbar (lower back) spine. Early on, patients were placed in rigid cervical collars and kept on uncomfortable, hard backboards until x-rays were performed, reviewed and it was determined to be "safe" to remove the cervical collar from the patient, and the patient from the backboard. Some physicians and other providers even waited for the radiologist to read the x-rays and send the report, making patients wait even longer on these hard and uncomfortable wood or hard plastic boards. On many occasions, patients were unnecessarily "forced" or "encouraged" to remain on these backboards for over an hour. With the advent of CT scans, the increased information obtained with CTs, and the speed and ease of obtaining them, some physicians jump directly to ordering CT scans of immobilized patients' spine.

During my emergency medicine residency, we reviewed much scientific and clinical literature and sometimes participated in research studies. We began to apply a simply protocol to determine if all these patients needed to have X-rays or whether we could release these patients from spinal immobilization without the need of x-rays and without putting the patient at any additional risk i.e. causing any unwanted complication including paralysis. This protocol consisted of taking a detailed and specific history and performing a proper physical exam. If the patient met the protocol criteria such as being awake and alert with no distracting injuries i.e. broken bone, known injury or other reasons for the patient to not be able to ordinarily feel pain i.e. under the influence of alcohol or medications, previous stroke, etc., the emergency physician would ask the patient perform certain range of motions with their neck so long as the patient developed no pain or problems. If the immobilized patient had no pain, met the criteria and was able to perform all the movements without causing any pain, the emergency physician would remove the rigid cervical collar from the patient and the patient would be removed from the backboard. We called this "clinically clearing" the patient's cervical spine. It was based on clinical trials that had been done and published in credible medical literature. No imaging was performed or deemed necessary so long as the patient met the protocol criteria. When there was any doubt, the patient had pain or pain with movement, had distracting injuries or was unable to meet the criteria, the physician is free to order whatever he or she felt was clinically necessary i.e. X-ray, CT or even MRI. The point is order what is necessary and avoid unnecessary tests that do not add any value or benefit to the patient's care.

Many paramedics thought this was crazy and some even criticized the practice. Perhaps they felt insulted or offended that physicians were removing cervical collars (c-collars) and removing patients from backboards without doing any x-rays after they had spent much time and efforts immobilizing the patient before transporting the patient to the ER. Patients often reported that the paramedics told them that they could have a broken neck and needed to have x-rays. Often patients would ask why they had to be on such an uncomfortable board for so long when they were taken off without any x-rays. Physicians would defend the paramedics and explain to patients that first responders were being careful and did not want to take any chances. I believe paramedics were trying to do their best. There was little benefit to criticizing them, especially in front of a patient. In the rare chance a paramedic acted in a manner that was inappropriate, it was be reasonable to pull the paramedic aside and speak with them in private. Often, this was a great opportunity to understand their logic and reasoning and sometimes a good teaching opportunity. Either way, it built a better working relationship with them as they appreciated the feedback and the fact that a physician was willing to take the time to speak with them in order to teach or help them. Unfortunately, many doctors and nurses criticize paramedics for various things. I see little benefit in criticizing someone for doing what they believe is right or someone who is trying to help. I am critical of those who complain about them who are not willing to take the time to communicate with the paramedics or try to help them learn and do things better. Even worse, some criticize them in front of others, including the patient, which is not only embarrassing but can be detrimental to patient care, trust, and the patient experience.

Speaking of paramedics, c-collars and backboards, reminds me of a story I was told by one of the most admired attending physicians during my residency training. The way I recall the story is as follows. A patient was brought in by EMS (emergency medical services i.e. ambulance) in full spinal immobilization i.e. c-collar and on a backboard. The patient was strapped down with belts and his head was taped so it could not move. This is the proper way to immobilize someone if you suspect a spinal injury may exist. It also is used if there is a concern that a patient at risk may try to remove themselves from the immobilization and potentially cause themselves harm i.e. injured and intoxicated. The patient in the story was inebriated and yelling. The report given to the ER staff was that the patient was involved in a motor vehicle collision (MVC) with moderate damage to the vehicle. The patient had been drinking and was immobilized at the scene and transported to the ER. All vital signs were normal. His exam revealed no obvious injuries, but the patient had slurred speech.

The paramedics kidnapped this poor guy who was only trying to be a Good Samaritan

When the emergency physician examined the patient and took the history from the patient, the patient told a very different story. The patient's version was verified by a friend that later arrived at the ER. As it turns out, the patient who was involved in a car accident was not in a car accident at all. The patient had been drinking at a bar. When he was leaving the bar and headed to his car, the patient heard a loud crash which was caused by a car striking another car or pole (this part of the story was not clear) across the street from the bar in which he was leaving. To be a Good Samaritan, the patient walked over to the car involved in the accident to see if there was anyone injured or needed assistance. It took him a few minutes to get to the scene from the bar parking lot and was looking around when the paramedics arrived. A few moments later, the paramedics told him to lay down and then they taped and strapped him down. The patient reported that he told the paramedics he was not in the car. The man asked to be removed from the cervical collar and hard backboard, but the paramedics did not comply. The man states that the paramedics told him that he could have a broken neck and they did not want anything bad to happen to him. Much of the patient's story was confirmed by someone who was at the bar with him and was in the bar parking lot with him when the accident occurred. It was verified that he had walked to the scene of the accident after the accident occurred.

As it turns out, the car may have been stolen and the occupants of the vehicle were able to get out of the car and fled the scene. That explained why no one else was at the scene of the accident when the paramedics arrived. The paramedics assumed he must have been the driver since there was no one else at the accident scene, and was probably denying driving so he would not get in trouble for drunk driving. The patient had been drinking, he did not deny that. That explains why there was the smell of alcohol on his breath and the slurred speech. His story explained the lack of injuries and was verified by others including the police who investigated the accident. Many poked fun at the paramedics who immobilized the man. The physician laughed about it and said the paramedics kidnapped this poor guy who was only trying to be a Good Samaritan.

EMS companies used to instruct paramedics to put people involved in car accidents, and who had fallen, in c-collars and on backboards regardless of the circumstances or the mechanism of injury. Some question the motives of ambulance companies that the paramedics worked for. Were they instructing their paramedics to immobilize all of these people involved in motor vehicle accidents (MVA), now often referred to as a motor vehicle collision (MVC), no matter how minor, out of concern for the car occupants, because they did not trust the judgment of the paramedics or because the ambulance company could bill a higher charge if patients were immobilized? I will hold judgment, but it is something worthy of consideration.

Until recently, many nurses and physicians in emergency departments outside of academic teaching facilities were uncomfortable with the practice of clinically clearing immobilized patients and did not follow the practice i.e. removing patients from spinal immobilization without first obtaining x-rays. Some called this practice stupid and ridiculed those who practiced quality emergency medicine that was evidenced based and taught in emergency medicine residency training. It has been over 20 years since my residency program has been "clinically clearing" cervical spines (neck) without imaging and still today, many still insist on getting an x-ray or even a CT scan before they will clear a cervical spine even though others clinically clear the spine without a single x-ray or CT. Many of these physicians and non-physician providers are not residency trained in emergency medicine. I am not aware of a single patient who had their cervical spine properly clinically cleared who had a bad outcome as a result of not getting the imaging by the emergency physician. One drawback of clinically clearing a cervical spine is many say the physician is taking a risk by not doing the test. But the clinical data shows that x-rays or other imaging are not necessary on patients who meet certain "clearance" criteria and allows the clinician to "clinically" clear the patient's cervical spine. The MD or NPP must accept responsibility, know what is supported by clinical evidence and be confident in their diagnostic and clinical ability to practice standard of care medicine. Another drawback is that the physician or NPP must ask the right questions and assess the patient properly; something that may take more of the physician's or NPP's time than to simply order an X-ray or CT scan of every patient who comes in immobilized. Substituting a test or image for a thorough history and physical exam is not advisable and not what many would consider practicing "good medicine." The irony is fractures and "unstable" injuries of the spine can be missed on X-rays. Even more important than an X-ray is good clinical skills and understanding mechanism of injuries and having a high degree of suspicion which is taught and emphasized in emergency medicine residency programs and using good judgment and common sense.

Children who receive numerous CT scans can have the same incidence of cancer during their lifetime as children who survived the atomic bomb in Hiroshima

Many patients wind up getting X-rays and CT scans that often are not needed. The need can be determined with a thorough history and physical exam rather than automatically ordering the X-rays, CT scans, labs or other various diagnostic tests. Some physicians are guilty of doing this. It could be that they are not convinced that clinically clearing a spine can be done without imaging even though the data supports that it can be safely done. It could be that physicians feel they need objective "proof" in the event there is a lawsuit and want to protect themselves i.e. defensive medicine. It could be that the physician is not confident in his or her ability to take an accurate history, perform a thorough physical exam and apply the appropriate protocol. It could be that the physician believes it saves time to order the study and not have to do as thorough of a physical exam. It could be the physician did not train in emergency medicine and thus lacks the training, knowledge or confidence to properly evaluate patients without "testing." It may be that the physician is lazy and doesn't want to take the time or do a thorough job. As I later learned, it could be that the physician is encouraged to maximize the amount billed to the patient thus increasing the amount that could be charged by the physician or staffing company. It could be because the patient requests it. It could be because somehow it provides the physician, patient or patient's family peace of mind. It could be any one of these or other reasons or it could be a combination of any of them. The point is that the current healthcare system is not the best it could be. The way medicine is practiced is not necessarily what is based on science, research, an understanding of medicine or common sense. It also demonstrates that the current healthcare system has incentives and disincentives that are not necessarily aligned with what is best for the patient.

Many patients end up getting many x-rays and/or CT scans and the accompanying radiation associated with them. This exposure could potentially add to the risk of later developing different forms of cancer. This is a whole other conversation, but the point is that if the test is not necessary or not going to change the treatment or outcome, why get it? What value does it add? For some reason, some people, including those in healthcare, feel more certain or comfortable if a "test" is done. Unfortunately, these people do not realize that tests are not perfect and have false negative and false positives associated. They may not understand the potential risks or consequences associated with these "tests.'

Radiation exposure is just one example. Not only does it potentially harm the patient, particularly children, by exposing them to avoidable radiation, but it is also expensive. Imaging can add hundreds to thousands of dollars to the emergency bill and not change outcome or treatments. So, this adds to the costs of healthcare significantly and it adds little to no value to someone's actual health.

Later I discovered that physician who ordered x-rays on patients were allowed to bill a higher level of service for the same type of patient presenting with the same complaints compared to a physician who clinically cleared the spine and treated spinally immobilized patients without ordering the expensive imaging studies. Payers will pay a higher charge for higher levels of service. Unfortunately, the way the system determines what level of service is often influenced by the number of tests ordered as opposed to what is wrong with the patient or how the patient presents in the emergency room. In this scenario with all other things being equal, the emergency physician who ordered the imaging studies was able to charge over 50% more than the physician who did not order the expensive tests and achieved the same, or what one could argue better, results. Put another way, the current healthcare system incentivizes physicians to do expensive, potentially harmful tests that add little to no value to the patient's health without changing the treatment or patient outcomes. The current healthcare system penalizes physicians financially who spend time with patients, practice high quality evidence-based medicine and achieve the same outcomes without ordering expensive imaging studies that are potentially harmful to patients. This is a fundamental flaw in the current healthcare system and another example of something that prevents the healthcare system from being better or reaching its potential.

As with other parts of the current healthcare system, the best interest of the provider and the patient are not necessarily aligned and may contribute in part, to why our current healthcare system is broken, especially to younger patients who may get additional imaging during their life. The incentives and disincentives within our current healthcare system are not what they need to be to make our healthcare system better. As I have stated, great healthcare involves keeping people healthy now and in the long term. Yes, it involves helping the sick or injured getting well again. But keeping people from getting sick or injured to begin with is even better. Prevention of illness or injury and maintenance of good health should be the goal. Unfortunately, the current healthcare system does not properly reward physicians and other NPPs to adequately promote this. Instead, its rewards treatment of disease and illness over prevention. It rewards ordering expensive and sometimes harmful or clinically unnecessary tests. The current system rewards ordering X-rays, and CT scans that over time when ordered over and over, may significantly increase the risk of cancer. It has been said that at the high rate that CT scans are being ordered, specifically CT scans of the abdomen and pelvis, which could have the equivalent radiation dose to humans of about 500-1500 chest X-rays, the cancer risks are real. It is stated that a CT scan of the chest delivers about 7 millisieverts (mSv) which is the unit radiation is measured. As a reference, the average person is exposed to about 3mSv per year.[45] Some say if children receive numerous CT scans, the incidence of cancer during their lifetime could be as high as children who survived the atomic bomb in Hiroshima. According to WebMD, "the chance of getting a fatal cancer from any one CT scan is about 1 in 2,000."[46] Some patients may have numerous CT scans within a week. Some patients with chronic diseases or pain may get frequent CT scans which over time exposes them to more and more ionizing radiation and a higher cancer risk. There are patients that get dozens of CT scans in one year. This is not to say that one should never get a CT scan. It is just to point out that the scans are not without their own risks. One must consider the risks of the scan and the potential benefits of the information that the scan will reveal each time. There are risks of getting a CT scan and there are potential risks of not getting a CT scan i.e. missed diagnosis, delay in diagnosis, etc. Some physicians may be concerned about the threat of medical malpractice claims if a scan is not ordered and there is a bad outcome. This can "encourage" a physician to error on the side of scanning as opposed to trusting her clinical findings.

In a world where no one is sick or ill, many physicians would go broke or shut down their practices. Why? There is "no money" in medicine if no one is sick. While this is not entirely true, there is a lot of truth in the statement. If everyone were healthy, physicians would only make money in routine exams and preventative medicine. Currently, this is a small part of the income physicians make. Most of the physician income is in the testing, interpretation of tests, surgeries, and procedures, diagnosing and treatment of illness, disease, and injuries. Payment for prevention should be a much greater percentage. If it were, it would help encourage the prevention of illnesses that are much more costly, in dollars and in human suffering.

The average income for a primary care physician (PCP) is stated to be $156,226 per year according to a June 17, 2019 search of job hiring site

Indeed.com.[47] Of course, many PCPs can and do make much more depending on the zip code where they practice, the type of practice they have, the demographics of their patients and other factors. Ask various physicians how many people they can handle within their practice and you might get all sorts of numbers. Depending on the type of practice, requirements of each patient and preferences of the physician. Ranges from 300 to 5,000 are possible but for our example, we will use 2,000. Decades ago, it would be much higher but with more regulations, time consuming paperwork and non-user friendly electronic medical record requirements, productivity and efficiency, seems to have fallen considerably.

Using these numbers of $156,226/year and 2,000 patients in a PCP's practice, the PCP makes about $78.11 per patient that is within his/her practice per year. Of course, this is not typically how PCPs earn their living i.e. reimbursed under our current healthcare system, they typically earn money as patients within his practice require care and the PCP provides services. We calculate the income per patient as a reference point or basis so we can compare other models.

With the mindset of paying for health and not for illness or failure of health, we re-set the thinking towards a better healthcare system. The goal is to keep people healthy before they get sick. What if we offer PCPs a base amount of $200,000 to keep the patients in their practice healthy? And what if we pay them even more, say a bonus, if their patients are healthier than before and use up less healthcare dollars as a result? Perhaps a percentage of the savings that is achieved by keeping people healthy. Perhaps offering up to twice their base salary. Do you think PCPs would be interested and motivated to keep their patients even healthier than they are now? This does not mean physicians are bad and only concerned about money. Physicians are people too and many people are incentivized by rewarding good results. With physicians, these results are better patient outcomes or better health. PCP's would have more skin in the game and more incentive to be innovative, creative and go the extra mile to keep their patients healthier. The PCP will benefit and more importantly, the patient will benefit.

How should a system be designed to promote good health? Incentivize physicians and other NPPs for great healthcare and penalize or "disincentivize" physicians and NPPs for sub-optimal healthcare. For example, let's assume that a physician cares for 1000 patients in his/her practice instead of 2000. If they only have half of the patients, they should be able to spend twice the time with their patients. Let's assume that $10,000 in healthcare is spent on each patient each year. On 1000 patients, about $10,000,000 is spent on healthcare each year. Of that, let's assume that 10%-20% of that healthcare expense goes to physicians. The other $8-9,000,000 goes for tests, procedures, treatments and other expenses that are spent mostly on illness. Thus, each year approximately $1-2M currently goes to pay physicians for those 1000 patients, or about $1,000-$2,000 per patient. This is over-simplification, as there are many different types of physicians that the current healthcare dollar goes to pay. Currently, the PCP averages only $78.11 per patient. If the DCO pays the doctor a $200K base salary, or even $400K if the PCP keeps his patient population healthier and meets the goals, there is potential savings of $600K-$1.4M just in doctors' fees to the DCO employer. Doctors make more than they do under the current system and employers/employees save more, a win-win combination. This assumes that PCPs are taking care of half the patients they currently do and get paid well over twice what they currently get i.e. $200-$400 per patient vs. $78.11 per patient.

Physicians take an oath to do no harm; they sacrifice their young adult life and dedicate their remaining years to help people

Of course, we would also have disincentives on the PCP should the PCP's patients have worse health in the short or long term. What if we were willing to increase the potential income to $500,000 if they could supervise and manage their 1000 patients and keep them healthier, which in turn would lessen their need for expensive treatments? Bonus the physicians for good patient health. This is a good thing. Physicians work hard and provide a very important part of healthcare. They provide care and can help influence and impact health considerably. If a system were to reward physicians for keeping people healthier, what do you think doctors would do? It is very reasonable to assume they would spend much more time and energy coming up with ways to keep patients from getting sick to begin with: more effective education of patients, home checks, follow-up calls, preventative care, etc. This will likely result in patients requiring less testing, medications, treatments and referrals but having better care and health.

One may question if such an incentive could have a negative consequence? Could it tempt physicians to be slow to order testing or delay diagnosing a patient with an illness in order to meet some criteria and continue to "earn" their prevention of illness bonus? One could argue that some physicians may intentionally withhold treatment, testing and procedures in order to lower "expenses" for the purpose of increasing the physician bonus. This is a big criticism of the insurers in the current healthcare system. While this might be true in a minority of cases, the likelihood of it being as bad as the current healthcare system seem very low. Besides being unethical, immoral and contrary to what most every physician believes is right, the physician stands to lose plenty for such behavior including medical malpractice claims, loss of their medical license and even criminal charges resulting in imprisonment.

Doctors invest too much time and sacrifice too much to be so foolish to take these risks and not do right by their patients. Physicians take an oath to do no harm; they sacrifice their young adult life and dedicate their remaining years to help people, often sacrificing family time, vacations, and other opportunities important to them. Unlike insurers who have shareholders to answer to and openly admit to trying to maximize profits, physicians must answer to their patients, their conscious and to many, their God. They often have long relationships with their patients and want to see them well. This arrangement only strengthens the incentive to find innovative and effective ways to do so. As a patient, who would you trust more to make healthcare decisions for you, the physician of your choosing or a health insurance company?

It is hoped that that this would not be the case. Most physicians sacrifice a lot in order to become a physician, so they can help people. It would be unethical and go against the belief many hold that the best interests of the patient, is their highest priority. Second, even if a physician intentionally stooped to such behavior for the purpose of earning a bonus, it would only work in the short term. Once the diagnosis of a patient became apparent and if it is discovered that patients of a certain physician were misdiagnosed or diagnoses were delayed, that physician would fall below his peers and in the long run, and would be financially penalized.

If someone gets sick, there will be no additional financial incentive for the physician to treat that person. They will still be obligated to treat the illness, and ethically they will still want to, but they will not get paid any additional money. If the PCP does not provide quality treatment, the PCPs will be financially penalized. The potential money that the physician can make will be reduced when patients get ill and require treatments because the physician gets a percentage of the savings. As people get sick, there would be more costs, which means less savings, and thus less additional money for physician bonuses for good patient health.

In such an arrangement, the physician would essentially have a budget she can use to take the best care of a group of patients within her practice. One would expect the care to be better, faster and cost less overall. Better and faster because it removes a third party, the insurer, that adds little to no value to care and may delay or deny care. Lower cost because with better, faster care and physicians aligned financially with patients staying healthy and using less resources, there will be money left unspent that currently is spent diagnosing and treating illness and injuries. The savings could be enormous. One might think the savings would be the money currently paid to physicians that is being saved. While this is a good deal of money, the enormous savings would be with the other approximate 80% of the money paid to other players in the healthcare complex. The trillions of dollars spent on testing, imaging, hospitals, medications, procedures, treatment and other non-physician entities that could be reduced. While this money does not currently go to the physician, by incentivizing the physician to keep people healthy, it may change behaviors and the way healthcare is delivered that will result in savings in the non-physician expenses. Many of the tests, imaging studies, surgeries, procedures, treatments and care would be unnecessary if patients didn't get sick.

One subject that is often overlooked or not given as much importance as many believe it should, is diet. While this subject is starting to get more attention, we still have a long way to go. It makes sense to think that what we put into our bodies influences the overall health of the person who is putting it into their body. If one eats food that is healthy and all other things being equal, it is more likely that person will be healthier than someone who eats unhealthily. Of course, there are other factors i.e. genetics, lifestyle, exposures, etc. that affect health but all other things being equal, a healthier diet should lead to a better state of health than an unhealthy diet. One problem is many physicians know very little about diet and its effect on health. Physicians are not taught sufficiently, if at all, about diets and nutrition in medical school and residency. One could argue that what is taught may not be accurate and certainly is not conclusive or complete. Something as "simple" as diet could make a huge impact on our state of health. Diet and nutrition will be discussed in much greater detail in the Diet Section of the Chapter 10.

By making physicians accountable, penalizing them for poor care or poor "patient population health" and incentivizing them to make their patient population healthier, we infuse a very effective mechanism to encourage efficiency and effectiveness. Patients win by being healthier, the physicians benefit by knowing their patients are healthier, suffer less and are happier. In addition, the physician benefits financially and can provide more for her family, staff and community. Society and employers also benefit. Patients are healthier, happier and more likely to be able to work, be more productive and thus add more value to their employers' businesses and society.

Chapter 6 Talking Points:

- The great majority of healthcare costs are not paid to doctors, but occur as a result of what lab, imaging or testing they order and treatment or procedure they determine is necessary.
- Physicians are an important part of healthcare and can have a great impact on improving the healthcare system.
- Physicians should be rewarded for having healthier patients as opposed to how many tests, procedures, and treatments they perform.
- Better incentives and disincentives need to be created in order to create a healthcare system that rewards health and prevention of illness as opposed to treating illness.
- Physicians take an oath to do no harm and sacrifice years to study and care for patients. Insurance companies want to maximize profits for their shareholders. If your examining physician believes you need a test or treatment, but your insurance company refuses to authorize the test or treatment, who should we trust?

Chapter Seven:
CONTRACT MANAGEMENT GROUPS
STAFFING COMPANIES

Traditionally, medicine has had independent physicians who practice their specialty. Often, physicians who practice the same medical or surgical specialty will form groups and have a group practice i.e. Internal Medicine, Surgeons, Pediatricians, Emergency Physicians, OB/GYN, etc. By doing so, the physicians can share the expenses of having a practice, cover for one another's patients, share call and sometime negotiate better rates with payers for their services. There are certain benefits to having a larger group including cost savings. A good example of this is in emergency medicine.

The public may not realize this but most physicians who work in emergency departments are not employed by the hospitals in which they work. Hospitals contract with large staffing companies, a.k.a. Contract Management Groups (CMGs), to staff their ERs. These CMGs then contract with physicians and NPPs to work for the CMGs and staff the hospital ERs. Most physicians or NPPs are employed or work as independent contractors for CMGs who "own" the contract to provide emergency department coverage. These CMGs are often located in a different state than the hospital, and often majority owned by shareholders who are non-physicians. Many emergency department contracts across the country are owned by hedge funds and private equity groups.

Over the years, people realized there was a lot of money spent on healthcare and looked at ways to make money. In fairness, there is nothing wrong with making money, especially if one provides a valuable service and charges a fair amount for that service. Particularly if one does good for the public and those who help them provide that good or service that benefits the public. This is the concept behind benevolent capitalism I sometimes use.

Most physicians who work in emergency departments are not employed by the hospitals

Decades ago, there were many small independent physician groups that staffed emergency departments all over the country. Many only staffed one hospital's emergency department, some a few, but not many staffed hundreds. Seeing the opportunity, some groups merged or bought out other groups. This was the beginning of the CMGs. By having larger groups, there is an opportunity of lowering costs and thus raising profits. The CMGs would handle the administrative duties that physicians may want to avoid. The concept of doing things more efficiently or providing a valuable service is a good thing. By selling out, small groups could take a windfall (big payday) and could still practice medicine.

Large staffing companies could recruit easier, provide malpractice insurance cheaper, often negotiate more effectively and realize other benefits of "scale." Being larger often allows a company to do things at a lower cost or with less additional effort or expense that it might take for a small "mom and pop" physician group. That is the good part or at least is the argument CMGs may make. Now the bad. As with many things, what starts as a good idea or intention does not materialize, often goes too far or is abused. Let's use emergency medicine, ERs and emergency physicians as an example. Many believe CMGs extract too much value from the physicians, charge patients too much and may hire less qualified physicians and non-physicians, which are often less costly than emergency specialists, in order to maximize profits.

Ethical physicians, who want what is best for their

patients, co-workers and the staff who care for patients, point out the short comings of facilities where they work

One might argue that CMGs rather hire less qualified physicians and NPPs over better trained, ethical and qualified physicians in order to maximize profits and protect their staffing contracts. Ethical physicians may point out quality issues, bring up concerns regarding the manner emergency rooms (ERs) are staffed, fairness of pay, fairness of working conditions, or how CMGs may put corporate profits ahead of patient care. Such physicians may be concerning to the CMGs. These well-intentioned and ethical physicians can pose a risk to the CMGs maintaining lucrative contracts that generate millions, perhaps billions, of dollars in revenue. One could argue that CMGs rather have physicians and other workers simply show up and not "cause problems" so not to bring attention to the deficiencies that may exist in the workplace i.e. ER, even if it meant hiring lesser trained and qualified physicians that may bring harm to patients.

What some may consider to be "less desirable" physicians or NPPs, CMGs may choose to look the other way. If one takes it to an extreme, less qualified physicians with quality related issues in their past are not overlooked but may be preferred as they these "less desired" physicians may be less likely to complain about working conditions because these physicians may not have as many employment or practice options at other facilities.

One might argue that CMGs rather hire less qualified physicians and NPPs over better trained, ethical and qualified physicians in order to maximize profits and protect their staffing contracts

A physician's past may raise concerns about the quality of their care i.e.

judgments against them in malpractice lawsuits, bad patient outcomes, quality concerns, etc. I refer to these physicians as corporate "show up and shut up" workers meaning that these less qualified physician and NPPs who have fewer options try to avoid anything that brings attention to them and do what the CMGs want. They show up to work so the shift is covered and say nothing about patient quality, patient safety, staff safety, fairness or any other concerns out of fear that they could be terminated. If they are terminated, it would be more difficult for these "less desired" physician and NPPs to find a good job as compared to a better-trained, more experienced, well respected physician.

Ethical physicians with integrity, who want what is best for their patients, co-workers and the staff who care for patients, point out the short comings of facilities where they work. They may raise their concerns about the inadequacy of proper physician coverage in staffing models, the failure of safe supervision of less trained and inexperienced NPPs who may be caring for patients too complex for their training or ability, or the inability to provide the proper care needed in an emergency department because of the way CMGs staff ERs. It may not be popular to do so, but it is the right thing to do. While doing so may ultimately result in termination, these ethical physicians have many other choices for employment. While one may say that someone cannot be terminated for doing the right thing and pointing out quality or safety concerns, the reality is that CMGs, hospitals and others may look for or manufacture reasons to label these well-intentioned physicians as "disruptive" or problem physicians to find reasons to terminate them or make the work environment such that the physician leaves. If the CMGs allows any physician to point out quality issues and staffing concerns without "penalty," it could result in others speaking up and force the CMG to make changes that could cost more money to the CMG and lessen profits i.e. increasing coverage by increasing the staffing hours or coverage, increasing the level of staffing such as using emergency experts as opposed to non-specialists or non-physicians, etc.

Others believe that private equity and the "commoditization" of emergency medicine has hurt emergency medicine and has harmed patients and places the public at risk. This is contrary to benevolent capitalism. If true, this may be why capitalism is often criticized. Some abuse their position to maximize profits at the expense and to the detriment to those they should be helping. CMGs should do what is best for patients and the people who directly care for the patients i.e. physicians, NPPs, etc.

With time, it seems more and more physicians believe staffing companies are abusing their position and charge much more (CMGs keep higher percentage of revenue) than the value that they bring to the physician. Even some hospital administrators may be starting to reach this same conclusion. Perhaps they realize that CMGs are charging much more than any value that they might bring to the hospital or community.

The concept of staffing companies makes sense. If someone or some entity can do things better or more efficient and bring more value to healthcare than they charge for that service, that is usually a good thing. For physicians, the staffing company can handle all the administrative issues such as recruiting, credentialing, scheduling, billing, collections, payroll, malpractice insurance, etc. and allows the physician to "simply" focus on practicing medicine. This concept appeals to many physicians.

The commoditization of emergency medicine has hurt emergency medicine and patient care

For hospitals and their administrators, the staffing company gives the hospital administrator a single contact that can help with staffing a single department i.e. the ER, or multiple departments i.e. ER, ICU, hospitalist service, anesthesia, radiology etc. It allows the administrator to spend less time dealing directly with each department and be able to better predict the staffing coverage and costs. If an issue should arise in any department contracted out to a staffing company, the administrator does not typically directly involve themselves in resolving the matter but instead calls the staffing company to handle the matter and may specify what outcome they desire. The staffing company can act as an extra layer of protection for administrators. Administrators may avoid having to deal directly with the physicians who staff their hospitals and can have plausible deniability if there is pushback or fallout from hurting a physician or other healthcare provider's career, reputation or livelihood.

One issue that is a concern to physicians is CMGs often agree to terms that harm physicians' ability to defend themselves from wrongful termination or giving emergency physicians the same rights as other physicians on the hospital medical staff. CMGs may include restrictive clauses in the contracts they have physicians and NPPs sign. CMGs may not fight to allow physicians to have due process should a hospital administrator want to terminate a physician. One might argue, CMGs are more concerned with money and getting a hospital contract than the people who work for them and take care of the patients. CMGs do not seem concerned enough to protect the physicians or require the physicians who work for them to be treated as fair as any other physician at any given hospital. In a sense, one may say that physicians working for CMGs can be treated as "second class citizens." It is not uncommon that physicians who are contracted with CMGs do not have same right to have hearings, have due process or appeal certain decisions. It is my understanding that there have been times when the hospital has asked for a physician to be terminated because an administrator requests it. There may not be a quality care issue, but it does not matter. The CMG only seems concerned about keeping their hospital happy so it can continue to make money. CMGs sometimes "ask" physicians to resign, as opposed to defending the physician, in order to avoid upsetting an administrator or risking losing a contract that an administrator may threaten to pull. The CMG may offer to move the physician to a different contract; they may believe the physician did nothing wrong and that the physician is good. They may ask for a resignation, so they do not have to go through the hassle and fallout of firing a physician. The point is that it seems that the CMG will do whatever the hospital administrator wants to keep them happy so they can keep the ER, or other, contract and continue to make money. They value money over their dedicated physicians and workers who may not have done anything that warrants a firing, will not properly defend the physician, do not guarantee due process to the physician or give the physician a fair opportunity to defend themselves i.e. CMG physicians may not have same protection as other physicians on the medical staff. If true, one can understand why physicians would not want to work for CMGs.

Physicians may lose 20, 30, 40% or more of the revenue they generate because they work for a staffing company

There are many other downsides to staffing companies for physicians, administrators and the public. Often many of the administrative matters that physicians are promised to be rid of remain the physicians' problems and the staffing company leans on them to work more than the physician wants. The staffing company is unsuccessful in recruiting new physicians as expected and lean on the physicians who preceded the staffing company to recruit to the site. The picture that is sometimes painted to the physician that they only must show up and work and the staffing company will take care of the rest often turns out to be a fairy tale.

Physician income can be significantly impacted by staffing companies. While staffing companies often do not share certain financial information citing proprietary or trade secrets as a reason, it is believed that staffing companies keep a significant percentage of all revenue. Physicians may lose 20, 30, 40% or more of the revenue they generate as the "expenses or fees" they pay because they work for a staffing company. Although the physicians do not get a bill per se, the CMGs collect much more from the services of the physician than they pay the physician. Often taking 20-40% or more "off the top" from the revenues the physicians are responsible for generating. It could be said that one of the only proprietary or trade secrets that staffing companies have is the percentage that they take from the physician generating the revenue from the practice of medicine by that physician. Even if the staffing company did handle the administrative matters for the physician, the staffing company's "cut" seems excessive for these services. Of course, the staffing company hides this information from physicians for obvious reasons. Keeping physician in the dark has been a successful strategy for the CMGs so physicians do not realize how much of the revenue the physician is generating that the CMG takes. Add to this that the staffing company often fails to handle all the administrative duties as expected or hoped, it makes this cut seem even more excessive.

If people only knew how many ERs used CMG physicians, who are not emergency specialists, they may choose to go elsewhere for their care

To give an example, while serving as a medical director, our emergency department sometimes would use an outside staffing company i.e. locum, to provide a physician to cover shifts. Unfortunately, we could not properly screen or vet the physicians before they showed up for work. The CMG had agreements with certain companies to provide staffing when needed. Often, the physicians that were provided by the staffing company were not emergency medicine board-certified physicians. In addition, many of them turned out to be "problem" physicians. Some of these physicians may have been some of the nicest people but their ability and skill to practice emergency medicine at a high level was not very good. What I mean by this is that their level of care often did not meet the standard that was expected in a respectable emergency department or by someone who understood emergency medicine and was concerned about quality of care, outcomes and professionalism. In fairness, as a residency trained emergency medicine board certified emergency physician, my expectation was high. That is the whole idea of emergency medicine training is to raise the standard and provide the highest quality emergency care to emergency department patients. This is probably what the public expects and assumes is the case all the time. If the public only knew how many ERs used CMG physicians who were not specialists in emergency medicine, who are not be the most capable or who may pose risks to patient safety, people would be surprised and may choose to go elsewhere for their care.

Many of these staffing company physicians have a poor knowledge base, poor procedural skills, less than desired bedside manner, and often generate many complaints from the medical and nursing staff as well as from patients. The bottom line is that many of these physicians may pose a danger to patient safety and I certainly would not feel comfortable having them care for a family member of mine. Sometimes I would simply work the extra shifts instead of using these staffing company physicians. One reason was ethical. I wanted to assure a certain level of quality in our emergency department. A second ulterior motive was to avoid getting so many complaints that as medical director I would have to handle. Ironically, the staffing companies that supplied these physicians often charged more for their services than what emergency physicians were making at our emergency department working full time.

Staffing companies also sometimes interfere or influence how physicians practice medicine which is inappropriate and can be dangerous. I later learned that one of the physicians being provided by a staffing company was being paid less than 60% of what was being paid to the staffing company supplying him. The staffing company was taking about a 40% cut. This apparently is not an isolated case with staffing companies. According to an article in ED Quality Solutions, Inc., "physicians who have worked for CMGs say that profits often drive their policies and decision-making, with some CMGs taking as much as 40 percent off the top for their own gain."[48]

Many physicians who work in the emergency department live in the same community where they work. They work hard and are involved to make sure the care provided to the community is the best it can be. They are involved in various hospital committees or emergency quality improvement efforts that often take a considerable amount of time. This non-clinical time often goes unpaid. These are the "administrative" tasks that are necessary or helpful to have a good emergency department. The physicians are often doing it, not the staffing company. Yet, the staffing company is benefitting financially for administrative duties that it should be doing that it is not doing. So if the emergency physicians are willing to and are already doing all or many of the administrative duties, it makes even less sense to have a staffing company involved that siphons off so much of the revenue that the emergency physicians are generating and could be getting paid.

CMGs keep physicians in the dark

Another important point. When a doctor simply wants to work practicing medicine and not be involved in any of the administrative part of emergency medicine or does not live in the community in which the emergency department serves, that physician may not be engaged and is often not the best option for the patient or the community. They are more like "renters" as opposed to "owners" who may be less concerned with improving the "value" or quality of care in that emergency department. They may simply come in and work for a paycheck and nothing more. This is not to say they cannot or do not provide quality services. It simply means that they are less likely to "invest" additional time and effort, beyond what is required contractually, to improve the quality of care delivered by not only themselves but also others in the emergency department.

CMGs keep hospitals in the dark

As for the hospital, the staffing company concept benefits do not always materialize. The expectations are often not realized, and this is part of the reason why there is so much turnover in staffing companies. The irony is that when a hospital administrator fires, or does not renew a contract with, a staffing company, they often contract with another CMG that often has many of the same drawbacks as the previous staffing company.

Another big reason why the staffing company concept can be so bad for hospitals is hospital administrators are usually overpaying for the value or service they are getting. As mentioned with the staffing company that kept 40% of the revenue that the physician generated, hospitals may be paying high dollar amounts for staffing or other services from the CMG and getting mediocre quality physicians and services. Using the emergency department (ED) example. Emergency specialists are experts in emergency medicine and are considered the "gold standard."

According to the American Academy of Emergency Medicine (AAEM),

> "A specialist in emergency medicine is a physician who has achieved, through personal dedication and sacrifice, certification by either the American Board of Emergency Medicine (ABEM) or the American Osteopathic Board of Emergency Medicine (AOBEM)."[49]

According to the American College of Emergency Physicians policy statement of the "Definition of an Emergency Physician," ACEP's website states the following:

> "An emergency physician is defined as a physician who is certified (or eligible to be certified) by the American Board of Emergency Medicine (ABEM) or the American Osteopathic Board of Emergency Medicine (AOBEM) or an equivalent international certifying body recognized by ABEM or AOBEM in Emergency Medicine or Pediatric Emergency Medicine, or who is eligible for active membership in the American College of Emergency Physicians."[50]

This is an important point for the public to understand. These emergency physicians (EPs) are experts in the field of emergency medicine and are different from the doctors who are not EPs and happen to work in the emergency department. It amazes me how the public is unaware of the difference. While these non-EPs are doctors and may have worked in emergency departments and may or may not be board certified in some other specialty, they are not emergency specialists. If someone were to require brain surgery, one would expect someone trained in neurosurgery who is board certified in neurosurgery, not someone who is a pediatrician or board certified in family practice. So, why do people not demand care by a specialist in emergency medicine for patients who are emergency patients? Why do hospitals allow staffing companies to staff the hospital's emergency department with physicians and non-physicians who are not emergency physicians?

EPs, being specialists, command, and deserve, a higher price that just any other doctor who lacks the training, board certification and skill set that they do. Hospitals may be paying enough to staff with the gold standard emergency physician but once the staffing company takes its cut or profit margin, they may only be able to afford and hire less qualified, less capable physicians. Sometimes even non-physicians are used to provide care to emergency patients. The staffing company simply may hire any physician with a medical license, emergency medicine residency trained or not, board certified in emergency medicine or not, good bedside manner or not, good procedural skills or not, good knowledge base or not, physician or not, to staff the emergency department they are contracted to cover. One could argue the cheaper, the better as that leaves more money for the CMGs to profit. Hospitals sometime end up with physicians working in their emergency departments that are average or less than average or who may not be able to work elsewhere.

I have worked for numerous staffing companies throughout my career. One company hired and staffed numerous physicians who some may say are "questionable" as to whether they should be working in an emergency department in any capacity. Some of these physicians were physicians that while serving as a medical director, I had not hired, pulled off the schedule or had to "let them go." It was felt they did not meet the standard needed to safely staff an emergency department and achieve good results in terms of quality and service i.e. quality concerns, patient complaints, medical staff complaints, nursing complaints, lack of EM training, etc. Yet, the hospitals where they worked were paying the staffing company and allowing the staffing company to bill and collect similar amounts as they would with high caliber and quality emergency physicians.

The hospital often pays the staffing company a subsidy to staff its emergency department in addition to allowing the staffing company to bill for, collect and keep the revenue from the professional fees (physician charges) charged by the CMG, to patients, for the services of the physician. Even the hospital administrators who do not pay a subsidy and only allow the staffing company to bill, collect and keep the professional fees, this can be very lucrative at some hospitals and the hospital could actually charge the staffing for the right to provide emergency services at that hospital.

After getting more and more market share and control by buying out more and more emergency medicine physician groups, staffing companies have taken more control of emergency medicine away from the emergency physicians. This is not a good thing. In fact, it can be bad for not only the emergency physician but also for the patient and the public.

Staffing companies, a.k.a. CMGs, keep the public in the dark

Physicians are typically the most knowledgeable about what is best for their patients and have a professional and personal interest in providing the best quality care. Physicians spend most of their adult life sacrificing to become physicians and to care for the sick. It is what they have chosen for their life. It is not all about money. Yes, money is important and it is fair to be fairly paid for the hard work they perform and the valuable services they provide. EPs and the ED staff are the safety net for the communities in which they practice and work. EPs are best to determine what is best for patients and provide the best care to them. This is very different than staffing companies. Large staffing companies are often owned by investment companies, shareholders or private equity firms who answer to their masters, shareholders. They seem less concerned with patient care, best-quality staffing models or healthy work environments, their primary focus is profits and return of investment to their shareholder or investors. May not sound very kind because it isn't.

While some staffing companies may have offered benefits that outweighed the downside at one point, others question if these benefits exist or are as good as one might have thought. Others wonder if the staffing companies have gone too far and are causing more problems than good. It is reported that medical costs can go up when staffing companies are involved. Often much of the costs that are paid for medical care are not seen by the physicians who provide the medical service. Perhaps this is at least part of the reason why large staffing companies are being bought for hundreds of millions of dollars and have values in the billions of dollars.

Many hospitals do not require physicians to be residency trained or board certified in the specialty in which they practice. The public is kept in the dark regarding this fact

Remember, staffing companies are companies and do not provide care. It is the physicians and non-physician providers that see and treat patients. So, one must ask, what is the exact value of the staffing company? Are they worth what is being paid for them? Are staffing companies worth what hospitals are paying them? Do these companies bring more value to physicians than they take from the physicians? Have the staffing companies gone too far? Now that they are bought for high dollar amount, are they trying to find more ways to make more money to justify the amount spent to buy them? Are they sacrificing care, quality of care, proper handling of the people within medicine in order to increase revenue in order to justify their value?

Most physicians in the country are not eligible to sit for board certification in emergency medicine because they lack the required training. Yet, any licensed physician can work in an emergency department (ED) so long as the hospital will credential the physician to do so. Many hospitals do not require physicians to be residency trained or board certified in the specialty in which they practice. The public is kept in the dark regarding this fact. Hospitals and the staffing companies do not advertise this. They don't want the public to know that their hospital does not have or require all physicians staffing their emergency department and seeing emergency patients to be emergency specialists. Some hospitals have zero emergency specialists staffing their emergency department.

The public should be concerned. One assumes that if one goes to the emergency department, one will see a physician who is specially trained, knowledgeable and board certified in emergency medicine. As discussed, this is often not the case. Some have proposed that in order to be called an emergency department or in order to use the word "emergency" or "ER", the facility should be required to have a board-certified emergency physician on site in the emergency department 24 hours a day, 7 days a week. This seems reasonable. It would assure the public that a specially trained emergency physician, who has undergone special training and has passed the necessary requirements to be board certified in emergency medicine, is available to treat the public at any time day or night.

Staffing companies and hospitals may not favor such a requirement. If such a requirement is made, many hospital emergency departments across the country would be exposed and it would be obvious many hospital emergency departments would not quality to use the term "emergency." The public would be aware of the lack of emergency specialists available in our country's ERs. Ironically these hospitals and staffing companies charge the same charges for non-emergency physicians as they do for emergency physicians. Some have proposed requiring board certification in emergency medicine in order to work in an emergency department and in order to bill an emergency medicine charge to the government or insurance companies. Given the unfortunate nature of medicine and how private equity has infiltrated it and has such a strong influence on medicine, perhaps changing the requirements of reimbursement and affecting money may be the only way to have hospitals and staffing companies provide the most trained, knowledgeable and capable physicians staff emergency departments and provide high quality emergency medicine care to the public. Otherwise, there is a financial incentive to use lower cost physicians and non-physicians who may lack the training, certification, skill or ability of emergency specialists.

Staffing companies, hospitals and non-board-certified physicians who work in emergency departments may argue that there is a shortage in the market and that is the reason why they cannot staff using 100% emergency physicians. This argument is often heard especially in the rural setting. While it is true that there is a shortage of emergency physicians this should not change the fact that we should be transparent to the public so it will know and can make informed health related decisions.

Requiring hospitals to have board certified emergency physicians on site 24/7/365 in order to use the word "Emergency" or "ER" would remove confusion and incentivize hospitals to require staffing companies to hire emergency specialists

Regardless of the cause or the reason why a staffing company or hospital cannot provide the highest quality and residency trained emergency physicians, we still need to be honest and transparent with the public. Be very transparent and make it very easy to know whether your emergency department is fully staffed with emergency physicians (the gold standard) or not. Some have proposed designating emergency departments in different tiers or calling them something different. If a hospital and or staffing company cannot provide this level of staffing, they can still provide medical care it just cannot be called an emergency department. While this may seem harsh, it is simply being fair, honest and transparent to the public. Even if hospitals cannot staff with the best, they should still have the responsibility to be as honest and open to the public that they are supposed to serve. Regulators should require such transparency as a condition of hospital licensure.

Another benefit of requiring emergency specialists to staff emergency departments as a condition of being called an emergency department, an emergency room, ER or anything that may confuse the public is it would provide incentive for the staffing companies and hospitals to work towards getting to this optimal level of staffing. Making this a requirement might improve the staffing in emergency departments and ultimately may result in 100% of all hospitals having emergency specialists available to the public 24 hours a day 7 days a week.

It should also help hospitals be more successful. If one hospital stepped up and had 100% of its physicians in the emergency department be emergency specialists, the public might realize the significance of this high standard and choose to get their emergency care at that hospital over others. This should increase the revenue at that hospital and serve as an example to others to upgrade to 100% staffing with emergency specialists in their emergency department in order to compete. This would improve the staffing in the community, which is a good thing.

This is not intended as a knock or criticism to the many non-residency trained non-emergency board certified physicians who practice in emergency departments. Many of these physicians are hardworking and can provide reasonable or great care to emergency patients. However, if we are being honest I believe most physicians including those physicians who are currently not residency trained in emergency medicine would agree that under ideal situations, all other things being equal, having all physicians who treat patients in the emergency department be emergency medicine residency training is good for the public.

In fairness to hospital administrators, sometimes they are fooled or tricked by staffing companies. When negotiating staffing for their emergency departments, CMGs like to use the term providers instead of physicians. As discussed previously, the term provider is confusing and is often used by some to encompass physicians, both board-certified in emergency medicine and non-board certified in emergency medicine, physicians board certified in some other non-emergency specialty as well as nurse practitioners and physician assistants. Is this term still used to trick, fool or confuse hospital administrators, physicians, the medical staff and the public? So, when staffing companies speak with hospitals and talk about staffing their emergency departments, they will talk about staffing the proper staffing using the proper number of providers.

If one is not aware of what the term provider means, and allows the CMGs to confuse them, then the wording of the contract can be such that the staffing company can use non physicians to staff emergency departments in place of physicians without breaking the contract.

Emergency experts can pick up on certain nuances and important parts of the patient's history and make important diagnoses that non-emergency experts may miss.

The staffing company might argue that a non-physician is perfectly capable of taking care of less serious conditions and it makes sense to use a lower cost non-physician to treat something less serious .The staffing company will argue that the non-physician physician assistant or nurse practitioner is under the supervision of a physician and therefore the care will not be compromised. While in theory this makes sense and can be true if done properly, the unfortunate truth is that things don't always happen as one might hope or expect. The other important thing to consider is who is doing the supervision and is the supervision proper. If the physician supervising the non-physician provider working in the emergency department a physician or an emergency physician? This is important if we are concerned about providing appropriate emergency care. While some states allow nurse practitioners to practice independent of physicians, many states still require supervision by a licensed physician of nurse practitioners and non-physician providers. Even state legislatures understand that nurse practitioners and physician assistants go through a minimal amount of training when one compares it to the training of a physician i.e. medical school and residency. It is my understanding that nurse practitioners and physician assistants undergo their education and when they graduate and become licensed, they can practice as a nurse practitioner or physician assistant, but their training is not specific for any particular medical or surgical specialty. For example, one does not finish as a nurse practitioner specializing in emergency medicine or a physician assistant specializing in emergency medicine. In comparison, an emergency physician must first complete medical school which is 4 years of postgraduate training and then must complete a residency program specific to emergency medicine after becoming a doctor. Emergency medicine residents must complete a 3, or 4, year program with specific training in various medical disciplines such as medicine, surgery, critical care medicine, pediatrics, pediatric critical care, obstetrics and gynecology, emergency medicine and other specialties under the supervision of faculty who are emergency specialists. Many physicians who have undergone emergency medicine residency programs have spent up to 100 hours per week training and have been exposed to thousands or tens of thousands of patients before they complete their training. Even after completing medical school and a residency program, the physician must then pass a specialty exam specific to emergency medicine before they can become board certified in their specialty.

The concept of having an emergency physician oversee a non-physician providing care to low acuity patients with simple complaints is not necessarily a bad one. Others might argue there is no substitute of having an emergency specialist taking care of any ailment in the emergency department even the simple ones. Sometimes common and simple complaints that seem simple can turn out to be much more serious. If not properly trained or experienced and one lacks the knowledge or diagnostic ability, these more serious causes may be missed because they may not even be considered, and the patient will be harmed. For example, a child who is fussy or not acting as one might expect may be diagnosed as having colic or an upper respiratory infection when in fact could be showing signs of intussusception or meningitis. If the diagnosis is missed, the outcome could be catastrophic. Another example might be someone with a severe headache. A non-emergency expert may order a CT scan and if negative, treat the patient's pain and discharge him and miss a life- threatening subarachnoid hemorrhage that might have been caught by an emergency physician who performs a diagnostic lumbar puncture. Unless one is properly trained, possesses sufficient knowledge and experience, and can pick up on certain and often subtle findings, these and other serious diagnoses may be missed. Because of the way emergency experts are taught and trained to think in their emergency medicine residency programs, they can pick up on certain nuances and important parts of the patient's history and make important diagnoses that non-emergency experts may miss.

One might argue that if there were enough emergency physicians no matter how simple or complex the patient's complaint, an emergency physician should treat every patient in order to receive reimbursement as an emergency charge. But if we go along with the argument that there is a shortage and we must try to make the best use of our resources, it is not unreasonable to use non-physician extenders such as physician assistants and nurse practitioners to provide care so long as there is the appropriate supervision and ensure that these non-physician providers are providing quality care within their ability and scope of practice.

The problem with this concept is when the supervising physician is not an emergency physician, and if there is not proper supervision, which may often be the case. It all depends on how one defines supervision, who is supervising the non-physician providers and who determines what that supervision will be. For example, if the emergency physician who is working in the emergency department hires, trains and supervises the non-physician provider i.e. nurse practitioner or physician assistant in the emergency department, and determines what the staffing hours will be, then it seems more likely and reasonable that the non-physician provider may receive adequate supervision as determined by the supervising physician and patient care will not suffer. It is not unreasonable for that supervising physician to have some responsibility and liability for the patients that that NPP is seeing and treating. However, many emergency departments have non-emergency specialists supervising and have staffing models that are not determined by the physicians who are working in the emergency department onsite and supervising the NPPs. The physicians did not interview or participate in the hiring of the NPPs and do not know the knowledge base or ability level of the NPPs. Instead, EPs or non-emergency physicians may be supervising the non-physician providers who were hired by the CMGs. The number of physicians and NPPs working at any given time determined by staffing company personnel instead of the on-site physician. Neither of these are ideal for proper patient care, and could be a recipe for disaster. Even if the staffing company personnel are emergency physicians, it does not seem appropriate for them to determine what other physicians must do because they are not onsite nor personally supervising the NPPs. The onsite physicians who are supervising could be placed in an unsafe situation because of the staffing model, hours of physician and NPP coverage that someone else determined and put in place. The supervising physicians could be liable for malpractice claims and more concerning, patients could be at risk by not receiving proper care because the NPP was not properly supervised.

As an example, a small emergency department may have one physician who staffs the emergency department at any given time. A large emergency department may have 2, 3, 4, or more emergency physicians staffing at any given time because of the higher number of patients it treats. Let's use an example of an emergency department that might have 5 emergency physicians staffing the emergency department at any given time. A staffing company may come to a hospital and tell them that they can staff their emergency department for less money than their current private group of emergency physicians who staff the hospital or may offer the hospital some other perk i.e. helping hospital coders and billing bill more effectively. Many hospital administrators are always looking for ways to save money or increase revenue and may be willing to make a change in hopes of improving the bottom line of the hospital.

Without going into a long discussion, some hospitals pay a subsidy to emergency groups in order to staff emergency departments because the physicians billing alone cannot cover the costs of the staffing of the emergency department. Often, there is a high rate of uninsured or under insured patients who come to the ER. Having said this, a hospital administrator may allow staffing company X to come in and provide emergency staffing for the hospital. Staffing company X realizes that physicians, particularly emergency specialists typically cost more to hire than NPPs such as physician assistants or nurse practitioners.

Some hospital administrators may not be savvy enough to catch the "bait and switch" of the CMGs

In order to maximize profits, the staffing company will change the staffing model from having 5 emergency physicians at any given time and may decrease the number of EPs to four instead. By doing so the staffing company saves 20%. The four remaining EPs now must see 25% more patients and may be overworked or may have to cut corners in order to see all the patients. This is not good for patients or the community. This allows less time to examine, treat and spend with each patient. This is not a good thing for the hospital either. The staffing company is more than happy to do so because they're making considerably more money by lowering the staffing level. They may likely have about the same revenue, but they have lowered their staffing costs by 20%. It is possible that the staffing company will continue to do this so long as they are able to get away with it. Now let's assume that the physicians who remain complain enough or threaten to leave, or that the hospital complains about long waits or that patient care is suffering. The hospital may tell the staffing company that they didn't think that the staffing company was simply just going to lower the staffing level. The hospital could threaten to pull the contract with the CMG. To respond, the staffing company states they will investigate it and adjust. The CMG now decides in order to increase staffing they will now bring on 2 non-physician providers. The CMG now comes back to the hospital and tells them that they have heard the hospital's concerns and are responding to them. The staffing company will boast that they're providing even more "providers" now than there were before they started staffing. They will tell the hospital they now have 6 providers instead of the 5 providers that were staff prior to staffing company X and try to spin this as an improvement. Some hospital administrators buy into this argument and are satisfied. The hospital administrator may not realize that the CMG is using NPPs to staff their emergency department or that there may not be proper physician supervision of the NPPs. Even with this staffing model, the staffing company is happy because they can pay less with four physicians and two non-physicians then with five emergency physicians.

Staffing companies are always looking at ways to increase their profits whether by increasing revenue or decreasing costs or both. So now staffing company X decides they will decrease the number of physicians again. This time they've decided to decrease the number of physicians to 2 and increase the number of non-physician extenders to 4. This way staffing company X can tell the hospital that they have the same number of providers and are able to provide care to the emergency patients at a lower cost to the hospital i.e. a lower or no subsidy compared with the subsidy that would have to be paid with six emergency physicians. Staffing company X will point out that even with this model of two EPs and four NPPs (six "providers"), the hospital is better off than they were before staffing company X came when they only had five providers. Again, the staffing company batches physicians and non-physicians together and calling them providers instead of identifying them by their degree, level of education or training. While there are hospital administrators who are quite savvy and understand the value of a physician, particularly emergency specialists versus a non-emergency physician or a NPP, some hospital administrators may not be savvy enough to catch the "bait and switch" of the CMGs. Some may not understand the difference or may look the other way because of the cost savings. Even though it may affect patient care or cause members of the medical staff to complain, many hospital administrators are so concerned about costs that they are willing to, or feel they must, sacrifice the quality of care in order to "afford" coverage of their emergency department. Many administrators do not understand how to accurately measure quality of care and justify the diluted type of staffing models or calculate the costs and liability associated with not staffing with emergency specialists.

Now let's look at how the staffing model affects quality of care and non-physician oversight. Initially in this example there were 5 emergency physicians providing care to the emergency patients. Each patient who presented to the emergency department would be seen by an emergency physician. With the new staffing model of two emergency physicians and 4 NPPs, many emergency patients now are not seen by emergency physicians. The two emergency physicians are unable to see the patients that they are seeing primarily and then go see the patients that the four NPPs are seeing. It is not reasonable to expect a physician to be able to see 2 or 3 patients an hour themselves and then see an additional 2 to 4 patients per hour that the non-physician providers are seeing and complete the time consuming medical charting, discussions and other responsibilities they have to perform. Yet this is the type of situation that many staffing companies might put physicians in. Such a situation puts patients at risk as they may not be receiving quality care or the same standard of care that the emergency physician would provide. Certain conditions or diagnosis may be missed because the NPP is seeing, treating and discharging the emergency patient without the emergency physician seeing the patient and often not even knowing that the patient was ever in the emergency department. This is not proper supervision and not a good or safe way to provide patient care.

There are many factors that determine the safe number of patients a physician can safely see per hour of work in the ER including but not limited to:

- Physician's ability
- Patient acuity-"sicker" patients often take more time
- Nursing and support staff
- Availability of beds in hospital
- Speed of ancillary services i.e. lab, imaging, ultrasound
- Efficiency of ER
- Support of medical staff
- Hospital requirements
- Responsibilities of EPs

Many believe if a physician is required to see more than 2 patients per hour on average, if patients are relatively ill, that physician is relatively busy and has plenty of responsibility to provide proper treatment, communicate to the ER staff, document in the cumbersome electronic medical records, speak to on-call or primary physicians, write orders and do all the other things that are involved with properly caring for a patient. Now going back to the example where there may be 2 physicians and 4 NPPs. If the physician is already seeing 2 patients per hour on average, they may not have the reserve or "bandwidth" to be able to see, or properly supervise the care for, the 2-4 additional patients per hour that the NPPs are seeing. In this case the physician is not expected to oversee the care for 2 patients per hour but expected to be responsible for 4-6 patients per hour. This is a very dangerous practice environment that will likely not end well. It is hard for the physician to know how serious these patients may be without personally examining these patients. Problem is the staffing models may not allow the physicians the time to be able to properly see all the patients that need to be seen.

According to the American Academy of Emergency Medicine (AAEM)[51]
- Every individual should have unencumbered access to quality emergency care provided by a specialist in emergency medicine.
- The practice of emergency medicine is best conducted by a specialist in emergency medicine.
- A specialist in emergency medicine is a physician who has achieved, through personal dedication and sacrifice, certification by either the American Board of Emergency Medicine (ABEM) or the American Osteopathic Board of Emergency Medicine (AOBEM).
- The personal and professional welfare of the individual specialist in emergency medicine is a primary concern to the AAEM.
- The Academy supports fair and equitable practice environments necessary to allow the specialist in emergency medicine to deliver the highest quality of patient care. Such an environment includes provisions for due process and the absence of restrictive covenants.
- The Academy supports residency programs and graduate medical education, which are essential to the continued enrichment of emergency medicine, and to ensure a high quality of care for the patient.

These are some of AAEM's principles and they make a lot of sense. They allow emergency physicians to do what is best for patients, unrestricted and unduly influenced by "corporate medicine" such as staffing companies that may put profits ahead of the best patient care.

A CMG model can put the public at risk. Often the patient is unaware that they are not being seen by a physician. The public trusts or may assume that the hospital would not jeopardize their care and would have emergency physicians in the ER. When you ask patients after they leave an ER, they will often say they saw the doctor when in fact they never saw a physician. Given this lack of understanding the patient may not know to ask to see a physician because they believe they are seeing the physician when in fact it a NPP. Unfortunately, even though many NPPs may be intelligent hardworking and good, the fact is they do not have the training and often lack the knowledge and experience that emergency physicians possess. It is unfair to expect the NPPs to know everything an emergency physician knows, particularly with patients with significant illnesses and conditions. The public is also unaware and uninformed of the important difference between a doctor who works in the emergency department and an emergency physician. As mentioned earlier, emergency physicians are capable of picking up on some nuances and subtle findings that can be missed by others. This can be the key to making an accurate diagnosis and providing quality care and preventing bad outcomes. This is often what many don't appreciate or take for granted. As mentioned earlier, knowledgeable and experienced emergency experts can determine when the diagnosis is not as simple as it may seem to a non-emergency specialist or a non-physician provider. This can sometimes be the difference between making an accurate diagnosis that could potentially prevent a potentially serious or life-threatening outcome from happening. Another way of putting it, it can be the difference between life and death. It is sometimes hard for non-physicians or non-emergency specialists to recognize or appreciate these subtleties or appreciate the significance of some historical or physical findings. As such, patients can potentially suffer by not being seen by emergency physicians and because of the staffing model that can be imposed on the physicians who work for these CMGs because the hospitals have chosen to use CMGs to staff their emergency departments who may use unsafe staffing models.

Many patients believe they saw a doctor when in fact they never saw a physician

This staffing company model puts the physician at risk. Because the physician, who will be supervising the non-physician provider, is often encouraged or required to sign a form stating that he is the supervising or collaborating physician for the NPP, he or she can be liable for the care or lack of care that the NPP provides. In addition, physicians are often asked to sign an "attestation" that they have participated in the care of the patient or that they agree with the evaluation of, or the care that was provided to, the patient. The non-physician extender might see treat and discharge a patient without ever informing the physician of the patient's presence, discussing the patient complaint, patient treatment plan or other information regarding the patient. The physician may never know the patient was ever in the emergency department or may find out days or weeks later when the chart appears for the physician to sign. This is an unsafe practice and puts patients at risk. It also puts the physician at risk of liability claims i.e. malpractice. Even worse, it is possible that the physician only becomes aware of the patient that was previously seen by, treated and discharged by a NPP, when the physician is served notice of a medical malpractice lawsuit against him.

Some physicians may feel pressured to sign an attestation on a patient's chart that they did not see or agree with the evaluation, or care, of the patient that the NPP saw without involving the physician. One could argue that the physician would be committing fraud if they attested to something that is not true. It hardly seems fair that a NPP essentially practices independently, which may not even legally be allowed in some jurisdictions, yet the physician is held liable for a patient he or she was not informed about and had no opportunity to see, examine or discuss in order to provide appropriate care and prevent a possible bad outcome. It seems unfair and unreasonable for physicians to be liable for lack of proper supervision of NPPs when the physicians have little to no control as to the staffing model and how supervision is done. It is also unfair to make physicians feel pressured to attest to a chart in a manner that the physician feels is deceptive or not true, so a higher charge can be billed or for any other reason.

A staffing company model puts the non-physician provider at risk. I am not implying that the NPPs are trying to do a bad job or are bad people. In fact, the opposite is true. The NPPs are trying to do their best to help patients and to help the physician in the emergency department see and treat the many emergency patients. However, because emergency departments are often understaffed, the physicians who are working are often overwhelmed by the volume of patients in the emergency departments they work in due to the staffing models determined by the staffing companies. The NPPs try not to bother the physicians or realize that these physicians are overwhelmed and therefore may not discuss patients with the "supervising" physician. Instead the NPP may treat and discharge patients without the appropriate supervision. Ultimately if there is a bad outcome, the NPP feels bad because the patient did poorly. The NPP is exposed to malpractice because of failure to diagnose or treat.

This staffing company model puts hospitals at risk. Not only do physicians and NPPs get accused of malpractice but hospitals are hurt in two ways if there are bad outcomes. The first is hospitals are often sued for malpractice or liability for not providing appropriate care and treatment for patients. The second is the damage to their reputation. A hospital may be perceived as inferior or substandard because of the lawsuits or because its emergency department is not properly staffed with emergency specialists or at the proper staffing levels.

Finally, staffing company models can put the CMG at risk. If there are bad outcomes, the staffing company can be found liable and is often included in malpractice lawsuits. CMGs may have to pay out a substantial payment if they are found liable. However unlike with the physician or the NPP, staffing companies aren't personally affected as a physician and NPP might be. As a physician, the physician is personally hurt, and it can affect them professionally and for months or years because of their personal commitment to medicine and the patients they care for and treat. Unlike what some may say, malpractice is very personal. Physicians do their best to take care of patients and when there's a bad outcome and they're sued they are personally affected even if they did nothing wrong. Talk to any physician who has been sued, I believe most, if not all, will say it affected them personally. Even if the lawsuit is frivolous or the physician did nothing wrong, it causes much stress and harm to the physician. However staffing companies do not have the same personal investment. It appears all about money. Some argue staffing companies are willing to payout lawsuits and consider them as part of doing business. So long as the savings in staffing with a less costly non-emergency physician, or NPP, is more than the cost of the lawsuit, the staffing company comes out ahead. The CMG may view it as a win. CMGs are less likely to change their staffing model unless it becomes, or is perceived that it will later become, too costly to keep the status quo. Because it is often about money, or the bottom line, to the staffing company. They do not have the same personal connection with the patient that the physician does. The CMGs do not have the physician-patient relationship and do not feel the same personal sadness as a caring physician does when a patient does not do well. The staffing company is often not headquartered where the emergency department is located and lacks the same connection to the community as the local practicing physician. If a lawsuit is made, it is typically the supervising or collaborative physician who is named should there be a bad outcome, not the corporate CEO or medical officer.

To be clear, there can be benefits from utilizing staffing companies and not all CMGs are necessarily bad. CMGs may be able to use their recruiting resources to find physicians to come to a remote or "less desired" place to live. However, one must also look at the drawbacks in every case and determine if the value staffing companies bring justifies their fee, or percentage that they keep from the physician, the control they exert, the amount they charge hospitals and how they may negatively affect patient care, the medical staff, the hospital and the community the hospital serves.

A CMG may be able to use lessons learned from other locations to help other locations avoid mistakes made elsewhere, etc. This discussion is intended to point out some of the many downsides that are often overlooked, not realized or neglected by hospital administrators and the public. Hopefully, CMG decision makers will realize that there are consequences to the status quo; they can make healthcare great again by doing what is best for patients and those who directly care for the patients, not just putting money ahead of people. Ironically, if CMGs put patients and those who care for patients first, if done properly, things will fall into place, and CMGs could make more money in the long run. Quite honestly, just about anyone within the healthcare complex stands to benefit from incorporating this concept.

Their perceived value would likely increase. CMGs may likely secure more contracts, increase their revenue, have greater loyalty and less turnover of their physicians and other non-physician employees and contractors and be sued less. Patients might choose where they go based on the CMG that staffs the facility.

Each situation is unique in some regard so hospital administrators, physicians and NPPs need to make the most-informed decisions for themselves and more importantly, for their patients and the communities they serve.

I have used hypothetical examples for emergency departments as I am most familiar with emergency medicine. Yet similar concerns are present for staffing outside of the emergency department. Many CMGs also staff radiology departments with radiologists, hospitals with hospitalists, operating rooms with anesthesiologists and even intensive care units with intensivists. Many of these other groups of physicians also face challenges and can be put at risk as can their patients because of the staffing models that staffing companies dictate to the physicians practicing their specialty and the oversight they are expected to provide even though the staffing model that the staffing company determines or dictates may not be adequate or appropriate. As there can be risks in emergency medicine, the same concerns can apply to these other specialties and areas of medicine. Not only are physicians put in awkward, uncomfortable and unsafe predicaments, but also the NPPs, hospitals, staffing companies and most importantly and concerning, the patients may suffer as a result.

Chapter 7 Talking Points:

- Not all physicians who work in the ER are emergency medicine residency trained board-certified emergency physicians. Many are not trained in emergency medicine and some ER patients are not ever seen by a physician
- Contract Management Groups (CMGs) may offer some benefits to hospitals and physicians but may have many drawbacks that are potentially harmful to physicians, hospitals and patients.
- Contract Management Groups (CMGs) often use non-emergency physicians that cost them less to hire but charge patients the same charge as for a board-certified emergency specialist.
- The public may not be aware that most physicians who work in the ER do not work for the hospital but are contracted by Contract Management Groups (CMGs)
- When patients get a bill from a physician after an ER visit, the emergency physician is often unaware of the amount billed and often has no idea of how much is collected in his or her name. It is common that CMGs collect the money and the doctor never sees how much is billed or collected under their name
- CMGs may keep up to 40% or more of what is collected for the services of the physician who treated you
- Hospitals that use CMGs to staff their ER often have staffing models that may threaten patient safety and be dangerous to patients.

Edward Shaheen, M.D.

Chapter Eight:

HOSPITALS

Hospitals are a very important part of the health care system. Hospitals, behind government, may be the second most inefficient entities on the planet. If administrators stopped worrying so much on money but instead focused on doing what was best for patients and what was best for the people who took care of patients, many of self-induced headaches and challenges they face would go away. I say this from my experience during my residency training and later as a practicing physician. Let me explain. During my specialty training, I wanted to learn as much as I could about medicine. I wanted to learn about the diseases, diagnosing illnesses and treating patients, caring for the person as well as treating the ailments the patients had. Learning about the business aspect of medicine was also important to understand i.e. charting, coding, billing, etc. During my residency training, I was very fortunate to be around many highly respected and talented physicians. I asked many questions and tried to learn from others, particularly those who I respect. Sometimes if the topic of money or billing came up, I would ask what they did or recommended to someone getting ready to start private practice. The message they gave me was consistent. They told me do what is best for the patient, document it well in the chart and the rest will take care of itself. I followed this advice then and continued to do so throughout my medical career and it has served me and my patients well.

I believe the advice I was given decades ago still applies today and not just to physicians. While being a hospital CEO may not be the same as being a physician, doing what is best for patients being paramount and things working out if properly documented is still very applicable. If administrators focused on efficiencies and doing innovative things instead of continuing to be wasteful and relying on the same habits and behaviors that got hospitals into trouble, the hospitals and their leaders would be better off. Examples of this occur in hospital emergency departments. One example, administrators often complain about the costs associated with emergency rooms: staffing with emergency physicians or non-emergency physicians, nurses, labs, etc. So, they cut back on staffing hours to lower costs, increase savings help the hospital's bottom line. Sounds reasonable but when one understands the complexities of the emergency department, this only makes things worse.

Do what is best for the patient, document it well in the chart and the rest will take care of itself

When hospitals cut nursing hours, often the hospital's bottom line suffers. Why? When there are less nurses, it takes longer for patients to be brought into rooms, longer for physician orders to be carried out and for patients that are discharged to be signed out and released from the emergency department. It takes longer for patients to be seen, treated and discharged which results in patients spending more time in the emergency department and occupying a bed that could be used for another patient that is waiting in the waiting room. Often patients waiting in the waiting room to be seen, leave without being treated resulting in many negative consequences.

One, the hospital has failed to serve the public. People who feel they have an emergency and come to the hospital's emergency room leave without ever being treated. Two, there are ethical, legal and liability issues with allowing patients to leave with a potential serious or life-threatening complaint. Three, the hospital's reputation can be damaged because it does not appropriately serve the community it is supposed to serve and does not treat people who come for help. Finally, it costs the hospital lots of money. The hospital charges patients a facility charge for being seen in the emergency department. This facility charge is significant and is "justified" by the fact that ERs must be open 24 hours a day, every day and it costs a lot to have equipment and staff available to handle most any emergency. In addition to this facility charge, the hospital charges cost more to patients for medications, supplies, lab tests, X-rays, imaging such as CT scans, ultrasound and MRI scans in addition to the facility charges. For every patient that leaves before being treated, the hospital cannot bill them for potentially hundreds to thousands of dollars of missed charges. It only takes one patient to leave without being seen and treated for a hospital to lose more revenue than it saves by cutting nursing staffing hours.

If administrators looked at the big picture, they would realize that the return on investment (ROI) of "investing" in hiring more nurses and expanding, not reducing, hours could actually improve revenues and profits in addition to doing the right things by patients and the community it serves. The same could be said about hospitals hiring staffing companies who utilize non-emergency physicians to staff emergency departments. It may seem like they are saving money but in the long run, they may be hurting their hospitals by losing out on potential revenue, hurting their name recognition, increasing themselves to liability from malpractice lawsuits, etc. In addition, when hospitals cut staffing or use less than optimally trained or qualified staff, there is often high staff turnover. Even administrators realize this can be very expensive to the hospital in terms of not only financial costs of hiring, training and reduced productivity but also errors, poor quality care and outcomes.

Administrators and others will push back when it is suggested that we should do what is best for patients and make that our primary focus. They may say money matters and it is naïve and ignorant to think otherwise. In our society money does matter. I am not saying it doesn't. The two are not mutually exclusive. What I am saying is the focus is often too focused on money itself and not enough effort on fixing the underlying problems that are contributing to a hospital's revenue and financial problems. As previously discussed, by doing what was best for patients and focusing on what patients want and need, we were able to add millions in revenues to the hospital. By understanding the concepts and ideas that are discussed in this book i.e. applying efficiencies, being patient-obsessed©, and successfully implementing them, hospitals can become more effective, more respected, and yes, more profitable.

Administrators can lower their stress level and can spend more time moving forward and doing greater things instead of being stuck in the past and dealing with all the problems that add no value and hurt their organizations. They can lead their teams and help their employees be better stewards to their customers, the patients. Administrators can fulfill what they hopefully want, to do good for the public and offer a great service at a fair price. If they implement innovative and better processes, the hospitals will be able to provide better care and services to the public. People will realize these benefits and these hospitals will be set apart from other hospitals who do not innovate. Ironically, if hospital administrators do successfully implement some of the ideas presented, and not spend so much time focusing on the money and distracting from their opportunity to truly be effective, the money will follow.

If hospitals were run in an efficient and effective manner, many things would fall into place

As mentioned, hospitals have a reputation of not being very innovative or efficient. Hospitals often do many things because that is the way they have done them for years. If you question why things are the way they are or suggest changing things, many hospital CEOs, administrators, and managers seem annoyed, frustrated, or insulted. They are not genuinely receptive to hearing new ideas with the intention of using these creative ideas to change. Decades ago, when hospitals were continually profitable, they could afford to take chances, deviate from the status quo, and make changes but their leaders did not make significant changes. Perhaps their leaders felt there was little incentive to do so. If they operated in the same manner, they would make money. The logic is why change or "rock the boat" if things are OK. They were making money. Why would an administrator listen to someone who advocates change and wants to implement innovative changes and risk failure? If the administrator was bold and brave enough to listen and implement innovative changes in order to improve healthcare and help patients and the community, and the changes were successful, the administrator might have received acknowledgement, been complimented and even given a small bonus. If the innovative changes were made and failed, the administrator would have likely been fired and lost a nice paying and often high-status job. The point is it was not in the best interest of the administrator to do what was best for patients and society. The benefits to the administrator, when taken into consideration, did not justify taking the risks associated with being innovative.

More recently, administrators have seemingly become receptive to change. One might say, some even seek out innovation and change. I would like to think this change in administrators' attitude and desire to make things better is because it is the right thing to do for patients and the communities the hospitals are meant to serve. Perhaps this is true with some of them. Let's remember, many of today's administrators are not the same people as the administrators, decades or just a few years ago. The skeptic in me makes me think that the "sudden" change in attitude and willingness and sometimes desire to be innovative and take chances may be because they must. They have little to no choice. Hospitals that are unwilling to change or remain how they were years ago will not survive. They lose money. Many have closed. They are forced to because if they don't, they will lose their job, either by being fired and replaced or because the hospital will no longer operate. No longer can the administrator rely on inertia and let things continue as they have before, and this is a good thing.

One would expect those in charge of hospitals to be the most knowledgeable, wise and efficient leaders in health care. One would believe CEO's and hospital administrators rise to their positions because of their knowledge and good performance. Often, this is not the case. Many hospital leaders end up in their position because "it is their turn" to be promoted or simply as a reward for being loyal, or associated with a hospital system, for a significant period and not because they have demonstrated superior leadership or the ability to innovate. One sometimes wonders if leaders become leaders because of their qualifications or because it is who they know, or they happen to be in the right place at the right time. One might argue people end up as a CEO or in a leadership position because they did well in their previous position, and this is often the case. So, when someone is promoted to a new position and they do not do well, they may be terminated, or they may end up in that position for a long period of time even though they fail to perform well as a hospital CEO or leader. This concept of promoting people to new jobs, as a reward for doing well, until they end up failing in their last position is sometimes referred to as promoting to incompetence i.e. a great nurse is promoted to become a mediocre charge nurse or a bad chief nursing officer (CNO). So now a good nurse is no longer providing great nursing care to patients but instead is mediocre or bad at supervising and leading all nurses. This occurs more than one might think and is a double whammy. It takes away a great worker in one position and makes them a less than ideal worker in another position often making that worker unhappy and those around them less than happy.

Promoting to incompetence is a bad practice

To be fair, I'm willing to give administrators the benefit of the doubt and believe they are qualified and doing their best. Even so, if one does not have the proper training, experience, knowledge and understanding of medicine and economics, as well as good judgment and a sense of right and wrong, the job can be especially challenging, and they are likely to fail. Having good organizational and communicating skills, an ability to understand people and situations and the ability to problem solve are valuable qualities that help make administrators successful. Without possessing these and other qualities, doing one's best often is not enough, and will result in outcomes that are less desirable than what patients and the public expect. Surrounding oneself with good people also helps. Administrators often answer to superiors and are too focused on numbers, figures and on the bottom line. Without the proper understanding of how patient care works, being able to connect with and lead individuals, possessing strong organizations and time management skills, creating a desirable workplace for those who take care of patients, understanding health care and how it can be different for each individual patient and all the many nuances associated with people, healthcare and the business of health care, administrators can be destined to fail by no fault of their own.

In fairness, hospitals are very large organizations with many moving parts. Administrators must deal with their bosses who are often individuals or corporations located in another part of the country. Administrators must deal with the financial constraints and limitations of their institution. Administrators must deal with the high cost of delivering health care including medications, equipment, labor and the many regulations that add additional costs to health care. In addition, there are many other factors including marketing, public relations, having to do what is politically correct, meeting with politicians to try to land grants and other funding, as well as the day-to-day operations, maintenance and repairs, labor issues, patient complaints, reimbursement, marketing, advertising, recruitment and retention of quality personnel, etc. Many administrators will tell you it is the hardest job they've ever done and no matter how hard they work there is more to do. Even the successful administrators who are well respected will admit that the job is very stressful and is very demanding.

It seems that if hospitals were run in an efficient and effective manner, everything would fall into place. Successful administrators may tell you just that. If one does their homework, understands the market, knows the strengths and limitations of their facility and people, they are better prepared and able to be successful. If administrators focus on doing what is best for the patient i.e. delivering the best patient care to every patient and doing the right thing by those who take care of patients, their job seems to be much easier and the results seem to be much better. This simple rule seems simple, yet many administrators fail to follow this simple roadmap. Instead, they lose sight, become too reactionary, lose focus and do not stick to well thought out strategy. They allow things to become too complicated and too confusing. Instead of focusing on what is best for the patient in the short and long term, administrators seem to focus more on the financials and often are short sighted. Administrators attempt to remain politically correct at the expense of doing what ultimately will result in what is best for patients, the hospital's long-term success and the community. Corners are cut in order to try and save money or increase revenue. While it is often done with good intentions, it all too often results in the opposite outcome of what is intended. These short-term savings often destroy the morale and loyalty of the committed staff who often determine the success or failure of a hospital, the value of the hospital's brand in the public's eye and reduce profits, particularly in the long term.

EMTALA requires any hospital that accepts governmental money to provide a medical screening exam to every patient who presents to the emergency department or hospital

Hospital administrators should try to avoid dictating or trying to influence how medicine is practiced. This makes sense that doctors should decide how to practice medicine within their expertise and not an administrator who has no medical background or very little background in medicine. Not only does this make sense from just a commonsense standpoint but this also makes sense from a patient care standpoint and from a medical legal standpoint. I will discuss one example but there are probably many others.

In the 1980s, the Emergency Medical Treatment and Labor Act known as EMTALA was passed. Essentially this law was meant to protect people when presenting to emergency departments. The EMTALA requires any hospital that accepts governmental money i.e. Medicare, Medicaid or Tricare insurance to provide a medical screening exam to every patient who presents to the emergency department. If someone has a medical emergency, the emergency department and associated hospital is required to treat the emergency within the capabilities of that facility regardless of the patient's ability to pay. In fact, the medical facility representatives are not even supposed to ask whether or not a person has insurance or how they plan on paying for the emergency department visit until the medical screening exam has been performed and it has been determined by a qualified medical worker that no medical emergency exists. EMTALA is more complicated than this but this is the main thrust of the law. Some may believe this law should not even need to be required as it makes sense and seems to be a naturally compassionate way of treating people. However there have been reports prior to this law that patients in need of medical attention including emergency treatment were denied treatment because of the lack of insurance or the ability to pay for their bill. For example, a woman in labor is told that because she has no insurance or ability to pay, she will not be seen at a facility even though that facility offers obstetric care.

During my residency training, I did the right thing i.e. what is best for the patient, and did not worry about the financial implications. This was the advice given to me by those I respected in training. I took it to heart then and have done so since and things have worked out well for me. I have passed these words of wisdom to emergency medicine residents and young physicians who ask for advice or why I have had a successful medical career. From a physician and public standpoint, this seems to be the best approach to take care of people. Unfortunately, sometimes hospital administrators or others in healthcare, particularly those who represent private equity or CMGs, sometimes seem to be more concerned with the bottom line than with patient care.

Emergency departments serve as a safety net to the public

Emergency departments are often called America's health safety net and for good reason. The public knows that no matter what, if they go to an emergency department, they will get at a minimum a medical screening exam and will receive treatment if they have a medical emergency even if they are poor, uninsured or homeless. The EMTALA law dictates this so long as the facilities accepts reimbursement from the government i.e. Medicare, Medicaid or Tricare insurance. If one spends time in a typical emergency department, they will discover that many patients who come to the emergency department for medical attention are poor and many are uninsured. If one talks to the billing or collection department, they will learn that many bills that are sent out come back unpaid or the envelopes are returned because of an incorrect or a non-existing address. The point is there are many emergency patients that are treated at a high expense that do not pay any money for the care provided. This is part of the reason ER bills are so high. The losses from these non-paying patients must be covered by profits from paying customers. If everyone paid, the charges could be much lower. From a business perspective, this is very bad and lessens any potential profit. If often causes some emergency departments to lose money and ultimately close, placing the community that it serves at risk. This is one reason why hospitals sometimes must pay subsidies to physicians or contract management groups in order to get physicians to work in their emergency departments. The collections from the billings sent to the patients, for the services they received in the emergency department performed by the physicians, is not enough to cover the costs of the physicians to work in the emergency department. Collections of emergency department bills can be extraordinarily low. One ER group I worked for allegedly collected only 16% of what they billed.

Forcing emergency departments to treat everyone regardless of their ability to pay has been a controversial topic to some for many years. Yet, the EMTALA law is a good one as it helps protect people and the public. As a physician, my priority is to care for patients and do the right thing by them. This is not only a priority of a physician it should be the priority of any kind and decent human being. Others say it is not fair to have to take care of the poor and not get paid for it. Others argue emergency charges are priced high enough where the losses that are incurred on the non-paying patients are subsidized by the amounts that are collected on the paying patients. But this is another story and can be discussed at another time. There is some validity to both sides.

Unfortunately, administrators of hospitals may sometimes try to influence physicians directly. Sometimes, administrators may try to influence staffing companies they hire to influence the emergency physicians to not work up uninsured emergency patients as thoroughly as they typically do. Hospitals may have policies or procedures to help "encourage" patients, who may not have insurance, to choose a different form of care instead of the emergency department. While there is nothing wrong with trying to encourage people to pursue a more appropriate form of care, once a patient presents to the emergency department, it is illegal to deny them emergency care or a medical screening evaluation because they may not have insurance or are unable to pay, i.e. EMTALA. It is fine to try to encourage patients to use resources in a better manner but only after one satisfies the law.

Hospital administrators should not try to persuade or convince emergency physicians to find ways not to admit Medicaid or uninsured patients or to circumvent the federal law

Trying to influence physicians to tell, direct or "encourage" patients to not receive care at the emergency department, especially based on their insurance status is, or may be viewed by some as, a way of circumventing and violating the EMTALA. I am told some administrators may outright instruct a staffing company or emergency physician to treat patients differently based on their payer status i.e. try to transfer patients with Medicaid or without insurance to another facility but keep and admit patients who have private insurance to their hospital. Hospitals have different procedures depending on whether a patient has health insurance or not. Other administrators may try to "encourage" emergency physicians to "discourage" noninsured patients from coming to the emergency department or to not admit Medicaid or uninsured patients to their hospital. In either case doing such things without fulfilling the requirements of the EMTALA is against the law.

Even most physicians understand the concept of having to be able to make money in order to have a sustainable model that will be healthy and able to exist so that emergency care can be provided to the public now, and in the future. Having said that, one must follow the law and not neglect those who require medical attention. What seems to make much more sense than trying to divert patients presenting to the emergency department or discouraging them from receiving care at a facility once they have already presented to the emergency department is to educate the public on their options before they ever seek care. Hospitals should market and advertise to help inform the public so they can make better informed decisions and seek care at the most appropriate facility. Many administrators are not willing to do this. Another idea is to provide some form of care or treatment that is available to these patients, so they will not ever have to have a medical emergency in the first place. Give people another option that they can choose to pursue instead of presenting to the emergency department. Because once they come to the emergency department, in fact once they set foot on hospital property, the EMTALA regulation specifically states the patient must receive a medical screening exam and should a medical emergency exist, must receive emergency services within that hospital's capabilities.

Hospital administrators would be much better off if they spent less time trying to persuade or convince emergency physicians to find ways not to admit Medicaid or uninsured patients or to circumvent the federal law, but instead spend their time looking for creative solutions to solve the problem of the homeless and uninsured being unable to get adequate care in a timely manner outside of the ER. While there are patients who do abuse the emergency department and use it as a convenient 24 hour a day medical clinic, many patients use it as a last resort because they have very few or no other options. Some might argue there are many programs including free clinics and other resources available to the public. While this is technically true, when one tries to utilize these services, there are many obstacles to receiving such care. Even when people follow the rules and do what they are told, they still may not get timely care. For example, the clinics accepting Medicaid may no longer be accepting patients. The clinic may allow the patient to make an appointment, but that appointment is cancelled before the appointment occurs and the patient must wait several weeks for the new appointment date. This is hardly an option when one requires medical care on an urgent basis, they cannot wait indefinitely to receive care. In addition, there is the risk that the providers who staff these facilities may not be physicians or may not be as qualified as physicians who only accept private insurance. Some argue that the physicians or non-physicians who treat Medicaid patients may treat the patients poorly because the physician and NPPs realize Medicaid patients have limited options or nowhere else to go if they are unhappy with the care or treatment.

There are some innovative ideas about ways to try to help lessen the burden on emergency departments that should only be used for emergency conditions and not as a 24 hour a day convenience. Hospital administrators should use the resources available to them and figure out ways that are most appropriate in their community in order to try to help solve the problem but still provide care to those who need it. Hospital administrators need to be knowledgeable and particularly knowledgeable about the business of health care or surround themselves with people who do. They need to be very knowledgeable about their business. One example is the need to know the specifics of the contracts they, or their predecessors, have signed and review them on a regular basis to make sure the agreements that they sign meet current market standards and pricing, and make sense. This is especially true for the smaller hospitals with less resources. For example, I was told about one small rural hospital that was losing money on a regular basis and was on the verge of going out of business. The CEO at that time, claimed he had done everything he knew how to do but was unable to turn the hospital around and ultimately stepped down after the hospital had lost millions of dollars "under his watch" and was approaching closure.

The hospital was put up for sale and ultimately taken over by a company who appointed a new CEO that I had the opportunity to speak with after he had taken over. I asked how things were going and he stated the hospital was no longer losing money but instead was actually quite profitable. He simply reviewed the contracts that were in place. Many of the contracts were old and outdated. The terms and pricing of these contracts that the hospital had agreed to were ridiculous. By reviewing the contracts and renegotiating the terms and the amounts on the contracts with various vendors i.e. pharmaceutical manufacturers, medical device makers and staffing companies, the administrator and his team were able to turn the hospital around and make millions of dollars of difference in the hospital's balance sheet. This did not even consider the many processes and deficiencies that could be improved upon to add to further gains. It appears the previous CEO did not know the basics. It appears he did not know "the numbers" or what was going on in his own hospital.

Another reason that hospital administrators fail or make bad decisions might be because they do not necessarily listen to others or take for granted the knowledge and the insight of others. Even administrators who have surrounded themselves with smart people can fail. Especially if they ignore what these smart and knowledgeable people have to say. Many of these people are not high profile or may not possess administrative credentials. It may be a doctor or a nurse. It may be a housekeeper or orderly. It may be a secretary or lab worker. It may be a patient or a family member of a patient. Administrators have access to some very brilliant and innovative minds, insightful people and many other resources that they take for granted or ignore. Again, I use EPs as an example. Emergency physicians for many years have offered suggestions to hospital administrators on ways to improve emergency departments, help improve the quality of care delivered in the emergency department, improve the efficiency of the emergency department and make it more profitable for the hospital. Emergency physicians and emergency directors suggested having a satellite laboratory located within the emergency department for point of care testing, testing that occurs at or near the point of care i.e. at patient's bedside, in the emergency department to speed up the process of obtaining lab results for emergency patients without delay. Emergency physicians suggested making waiting rooms more desirable, increasing staff to allow for better care and a better experience for emergency patients and improving the processes within the emergency department in order to decrease wait times and the time that patients had to spend in the emergency department. Emergency physicians wanted to make emergency departments "patient focused" decades ago. For decades physicians offered their opinions, but few administrators ever listened enough or were willing to act on emergency physician suggestions.

Hospital administrators sometimes listened and sometimes they did not listen, but they rarely ever made the changes that the emergency physicians had suggested or requested. Emergency departments were often labeled as money pits and big losers for the hospital. Administrators seem to overlook the fact that emergency departments were often the face of the hospital and were big money makers for the hospital. Emergency departments not only charged and collected money for emergency treatment but they generated a large portion of the hospital's total revenue because of all the hospital admissions that are generated through the emergency department, all the radiology testing that is done in the emergency department and all the laboratory studies that are done in the emergency department. Because of accounting methods hospitals use, credit is given to other departments for what is generated in the emergency department. For example:

- X-rays and CT imaging done in the emergency department is credited to the radiology department
- Lab studies ordered in the emergency department are credited to the laboratory
- Blood transfusions are credited to the blood bank
- Admissions generated in the emergency department are credited to the intensive care unit (ICU), medical unit, surgical unit, etc.

The point is that administrators mistakenly saw the emergency department as a negative for the hospitals instead of as an asset. And it was not one administrator, it was a common belief by many hospital administrators throughout the country. It was sometimes said that the "ER is the red-headed stepchild" of the hospital as it was often neglected and not taken seriously. Perhaps the hospital administrators didn't believe the emergency physicians, perhaps they didn't care or perhaps they did not make the change because they felt the emergency physicians and the public had little to no choice, so the hospital did not have to make improvements. Who knows?

Emergency physicians had little recourse. They didn't have the power or authority to implement changes unless they had the approval or permission of the hospital administrators and they could not practice emergency medicine anywhere except in a hospital. Only hospitals had emergency departments where emergency specialists could practice their specialty. Unlike other physicians who can open their own office and practice their specialty, emergency physicians could not just go and open an emergency department. Even if the emergency physician could afford or find financing for the venture, state laws did not allow for a non-hospital to operate an emergency department. This changed in recent years. Sometime in the past 20 years, some states changed their laws and allowed emergency centers to exist that were not owned by a hospital. Texas passed laws that may have been the most favorable. Non-hospitals, including emergency physicians, or anyone else who could meet the requirements, were able to own and operate them. This opportunity was jumped upon by business minded emergency physicians who opened freestanding emergency centers (FECs). These FECs blossomed all over and there are hundreds of them in Texas. Many emergency physicians left their hospital-based jobs and worked in FECs. The pay was better but most importantly, these places allowed them to control the way they practiced their specialty. Non-physicians, staffing companies and hospitals did not dictate how emergency physicians had to practice their specialty as they do in the traditional ERs that are located within hospitals. The FECs were also fun to work in. They were efficient, wait times were minimal and physicians felt heard and respected. Most importantly, patients loved them because they felt they received better care and service in FECs than they might in a traditional ER.

Hospital administrators seemed surprised and even shocked. They became upset how others were able to compete with them. They were even more upset because these new freestanding emergency centers, were successful and took many patients away from the traditional emergency departments particularly the insured patients that the hospital administrators cherished. These freestanding emergency centers, not owned by hospitals, turned many of their owners into millionaires. These freestanding emergency centers were able to pay the emergency physicians taking care of the patients in emergency centers as much as, or more than, emergency physicians who worked in traditional emergency departments. These freestanding emergency centers had emergency physicians making decisions on how the freestanding emergency centers should be run. If a new piece of equipment was needed or a change in some capital expenditure needed to be made these were often welcomed and implemented in short order. This was a drastic change from what emergency physicians were accustomed to having to ask, sometimes beg, hospital administrators for necessary equipment and changes and only be denied and disappointed.

Hospital administrators sometimes fail to listen to, or take for granted, the knowledge and the insight of others around them

The irony is many of the emergency physicians who ultimately went on to start and own freestanding emergency centers were not implementing anything drastically new other than the center itself. Many of the ideas and processes used in the emergency centers were ideas that were offered free of charge for years to hospital administrators in hopes of making the emergency departments within hospitals better. The problem is the hospital administrators did not listen to this valuable input or implement the changes. So, when the emergency physicians had their chance, they seized upon it and created emergency centers. The freestanding emergency centers advertised their convenience in close locations to residential areas. They offered snacks, drinks and conveniences in the waiting room. They hired enough people to make sure that service in the freestanding emergency center was superior, and they focused on patient care knowing that by doing what is best for the patient would attract patients and ultimately maximize their bottom line.

Patients do not know or care why it is faster, they just like it when they are seen quickly, treated kindly and feel special

In freestanding emergency centers, many patients were seen and treated much quicker than they would be in a traditional emergency department. Once placed in a room, often straight from the emergency waiting room without any wait, patients are often immediately seen by the emergency physician. Many of the freestanding emergency centers are staffed 100% by emergency specialists, whereas many traditional emergency department's still staff with non-emergency physicians and sometimes even non physicians. The operators of these FECs seem to understand the value of staffing with specialists in emergency medicine, not just any doctor with a medical license. These freestanding emergency centers have point of care testing, CT scanners, X Rays, ultrasound, and EKG availability all within the freestanding emergency center. Unlike bigger emergency departments contained within a hospital that must take labs to a different department in another part of the hospital and wait for results or send people to a radiology department and wait for results, FECs eliminate these inefficiencies that add no value to the patient or patient care. Often labs are performed and from the time the blood is drawn from the patient, the physician will have the result within minutes. Sometimes it may take hours in a traditional emergency department because of delays in transporting the lab specimen to the laboratory, the delay in the laboratory getting the specimen to the time that they batch lab specimens and/or put the specimen into the machine, the time that the lab is completed to the time that the laboratory technician records the results, and the time that the laboratory result is entered into the computer where it is available for the physician to see. The point is these freestanding emergency centers are more conducive to the efficient, expeditious and quality care of the patient than hospital-based emergency departments. The time it takes to treat patients is reduced. Patients do not know or care why it is faster, they just like it when they are seen quickly, treated kindly and feel special.

And the reasons why FECs are efficient and care is quick is because FECs followed the suggestions that emergency physicians, for years, have suggested to hospital administrators. These administrators missed a great opportunity because they did not listen to the people who knew emergency medicine. After it was obvious that these FECs were attracting many patients and a financial success and taking many of the insured patients that hospitals desired, hospital administrators began to make the changes that emergency physicians had suggested for years. Hospitals later copied the FEC model that emergency physicians helped pioneer. What is the saying? Imitation is the ultimate form of flattery.

As mentioned at the beginning of this chapter, hospitals are very inefficient. Often, they have many people doing many things that add little or no value to patient care or the bottom line. Often, people are paid to do things that may take away value from a hospital. As with the example of the hospital that was losing money that was turned around when a new CEO came in, reviewed and re-negotiated the contracts, many hospital administrators have little to no idea of exactly what people do, what they are paid and how much their efforts affect patient care and the bottom line. No wonder why so many administrators fail. It's hard to make good decisions without accurate information.

Patients come to the ER to see "the doctor"

One hospital in a southern state, where I worked, was losing millions of dollars annually not long after making millions in profits. After much efforts and convincing, the hospital allowed us to change some processes in the emergency department. The process of how patients were seen, eliminating waits, and the order in which things were done and empowering staff, it is reported the emergency department helped generate an additional $5,000,000 in hospital revenue in a single year. It was not that complicated. I spoke with patients, staff and just about anyone who had anything to do with the emergency department. When speaking to patients, common themes became obvious. Patients come to the ER to "see the doctor" and patients do not like to wait. When one looks at how things have traditionally been done and remain in effect at many ERs across the country, patients are made to "jump through many hoops" and made to wait before being allowed to see the doctor; the exact opposite of what people want. Patients who come to the ER:

1) Must register at the front desk
2) Wait to be called to be "triaged." Typically, a nurse will take the patient's vital signs and asks some medical questions related to the patient's complaint, reason for going to the ER. Triage is a

way to prioritize what patients must be seen immediately and which patients are able to wait with less chance of a deterioration of their condition.

3) Are triaged typically by a nurse
4) Wait to be called to an exam or treatment room
5) Are called and placed in an exam or treatment room
6) Wait in that treatment room for the ER nurse that will be caring for the patient in the "back"/treatment area
7) Be seen by the nurse
8) Wait for the doctor or NPP
9) See the physician or NPP
10) Wait for any tests that may be ordered by the physician or NPP to be performed i.e. blood drawn, X-rays or imaging performed, and wait for any treatments that may be ordered by the physician or NPP to be performed
11) Wait for the results of these tests
12) Wait for the physician or NPP to come back and explain the findings
13) Wait for the nurse to come provide discharge instructions and discharge the patient.

Patients say they come to the ER to "see the doctor," but we make them go through at least 7 steps before they see the doctor, if they ever see a doctor. This made no sense to me. This is something that has bothered me since my residency. Why do we make our patients go through so much before we give them what they want? I.e. to "see the doctor." The "customer service" in hospitals was terrible. Why don't we give patients what they want? I learned at a very young age, while growing up and spending so much of my childhood in our family restaurant during the 1970's and 1980's, when customers were scarce because people did not eat out very often, to give the customer what they wanted. Provide them a good product but even more importantly, provide them the best service. Give them a pleasant experience. Respect their time and show your appreciation of their business by respecting their time and doing what was best for them. By following this concept, our family restaurant was able to survive when many other restaurants were losing money and going out of business.

As a medical director, I championed the implementation of immediate bedding for patients. Instead of making people wait and go through a series of steps before they ever saw a doctor i.e. steps #1-#7 above, the patient was registered and then placed in a room. Sometimes patients were placed in rooms before they were even registered. I understood that many different people often had to do many different things related to the patient i.e. register them, nursing assessment, draw blood, take X-rays, etc. before they were ultimately discharged from the ER or admitted to the hospital but nothing stated that they had to be done in a certain sequence. Why did we have to only do one thing at a time and in a certain order? Why not do many of the required tasks concurrently instead of sequentially? Why not do what we can right now and only make the patient wait if that resource is not immediately available? It just made sense.

We can still provide quality care, even better care, if we allow the doctor or anyone else to see the patient as soon as possible so everything that needs to be done can be done in the shortest time possible. This is what patients want! Just ask them; I did. They want to see the doctor and do not like to wait remember. Even if the patient has a simple complaint and could wait in the waiting room without causing any harm, why make them wait? See them now, treat them and discharge them. They will be one less patient that has to wait when the ER gets slammed with emergency or critical patients. It will also make the patient have a good experience that he or she will remember the next time they, or a family member, seek medical care. It is good business to have people leave with a good experience rather than with a bad one.

Another reason for immediate bedding is that it helps the staff. As a physician, I may not be busy now when a patient with a non-serious complaint checks in and could be seen by me immediately and be discharged. If the patient is made to wait, because it is "not an emergency" or other reasons, by the time the patient is placed in a room, I may be busy with a cardiac, trauma or other critical patient and unable to leave that room to see the patient with a non-serious condition that was made to wait. I could be tied up with a critical patient for an hour or more. This concept applies for everyone else in the care team. Place the patient in a room, if any services are needed, as soon as that team member whose services are required is available, they can provide their service to the patient. This concept was what was in the best interest of the patient and as many learned, turned out to be in the staff's best interest. It improved our efficiency, allowed us to provide better care and see more people in less time than the previous process. This process helped us see more patients and made it seem less like work. Physicians and other ER staff did not seem as tired at the end of their shifts even though they saw more patients.

This process helped our emergency department cut patient wait times, reduced the number of patients who left the waiting room because of long wait times, decreased the number of patient and staff complaints and improved quality measures for our emergency department. This same process was implemented in another emergency department where I served as medical director and our emergency department was recognized for our success. We beat out all other hospitals within our healthcare system across the country.

The same hospital, used in my first example of the success of immediate bedding, did an audit of their staff and discovered that there were many on their payroll that did not have defined rolls. There were nurses receiving pay but not providing any patient care. The hospital administrators realized that they did not know what was going on in their own house. The hospital provided an incentive for many employees to leave in order to save money after they investigated their staff and the salaries that they were making and the services that they were providing.

An administrator has to know his limitations and the limitations of his hospital

Often hospitals have many administrative personnel. While there can be value in administrative personnel, it seems that many hospitals do a poor job of objectively knowing what is being done, quantifying how it affects care and quantifying how it affects the bottom line, both in terms of how it affects costs and revenue. Often hospital leaders fail to re-evaluate contracts, staffing models and other organizational policies and procedures frequent enough to make sure they make sense and are what is best for their patients, the people who take care of patients and the organization. This is a common mistake committed by government. This may be why both are so inefficient and are accused of wasting so much money. Many times, hospitals have committees and they meet and meet and meet. They discuss things over and over, but they do not seem to act upon the information they have spent so much time and effort to gather. If one is not going to act on information, why the heck would someone spend so much to gather it? It just doesn't make sense. I brought this very point up with administrators and they seemed upset. They did not have a good answer at the time and seemed shocked by how I dare ask such a question or point out what should have been obvious to anyone who uses common sense, good judgment and thinks logically.

Some hospital administrators have egos. To some degree this can be good, but it can also be a negative attribute. As Clint Eastwood's character Harry Callahan said in the 1973 movie *Magnum Force*[52], "A Man's got to Know His Limitations." So does a hospital or administrator. Some hospitals can do many things well, but many hospitals cannot. Instead of accepting this reality and doing what they do well and profitably, hospitals sometimes try to do too much and end up losing money and providing care inferior to what another hospital may be able to provide. This is not good for the hospitals and even worse, it is not what is best for the patient or the community the hospital is meant to serve.

Sometimes the opposite can be true. Sometimes hospitals only do certain things and their representatives will do their best to avoid caring for a patient. They will try to find any excuse to refuse accepting or treating a patient. An example of this is with hospital transfers. Going back to EMTALA, if an emergency patient at one hospital's ER needs care or treatment that the hospital cannot provide, EMTALA requires the nearest hospital that can provide the needed services to accept the patient without consideration of the patient's ability to pay or not. So if an ER physician calls the hospitalist (admitting doctor) at his/her hospital to admit a person with cellulitis (skin infection) who also happens to have chronic obstructive pulmonary disease (COPD), that hospitalist may refuse to admit the patient using the reason/excuse that there is not a pulmonologist Lung specialist) at the hospital in the event the patient needs one. This may seem reasonable if the patient is having severe problems breathing, likely to require intubation and mechanical ventilation (being placed on a ventilator) or will require aggressive pulmonary management. But even if the patient not having any problems breathing, their COPD is well controlled and the patient has never required being placed on a ventilator, some hospitalists may still refuse to admit such a patient because of the history of COPD. Add to this, COPD is a common condition and most hospitalists should be very familiar with, and capable of, treating COPD. This makes little sense. The patient will have to travel elsewhere to get care that could be provided at the hospital where the patient is currently located. This drive costs up unnecessarily, can be a significant inconvenience to the patient, the transferring hospital staff and the receiving hospital staff. This is not the "right" thing to do but can happen. Hospital administrators need to be more knowledgeable of what goes on in their hospital so they can make better informed and sensible decisions that will help others in their hospital do the right thing and what is in the best interest of the patients and communities they serve.

Along these same lines that some hospital administrators do not know what is going on in the hospitals they run, many hospital administrators would benefit from getting out of their corporate suite and interacting on a regular basis with patients and employees throughout their hospital and organization. Do "field research." One can learn a lot from seeing things for themselves. The term "a picture is worth a thousand words" applies. Going to the ER on a regular basis, up to the various floors, the ICU, radiology department, waiting rooms of various departments, cafeteria, registration, OR etc. Just go and watch, talk to people and patients, families, physicians and employees and listen. Administrators who are good at asking the right questions, listening and using good judgment can benefit enormously from doing field research. Some administrators might spend tens of thousands of dollars hiring consultants to tell them what is wrong with, or not going well at, their hospital when they can learn this valuable information on their own if they spent more time visiting the various areas of their hospitals and interacting with their staff and the people they serve. Administrators should spend at least 50% of their time in the hospital doing this. In addition to gaining lots of information and knowledge that will help administrators make better informed and hopefully better decisions, it can help build moral, respect and trust from the employees. It also helps the administrator have a better appreciation of their staff and all that they do. The more successful administrators have figured out the value and importance of such field research.

By talking to patients and the people who care for them, administrators will learn and better understand the challenges. They learn what is being done well and what could be done better. They will have the opportunity to ask those with firsthand knowledge for ideas that could help the administrator come up with solutions or improvements. This "costs" little to nothing but can be invaluable. Remember the emergency physician and ER example. Had the administrators listened to those emergency physicians, they could have made improvements in the hospitals and benefited from them instead of alienating the emergency physicians, giving incentives for smart, hard-working, resourceful and well-intentioned emergency physicians to leave and do their own thing when the opportunity presented itself and losing these "desired" emergency specialists to the freestanding emergency centers.

An administrator cannot be viewed as a hypocrite

Administrators need to establish a healthy culture, work environment and mission statement for the hospital. They must set the bar for what the expectations are for anyone associated with that hospital and/or organizations. Once set, the administrator needs to live up to and above the bar. The administrator must be a great example and a role model for everyone in the organization. An administrator cannot be viewed as a hypocrite, expecting others to sacrifice and place patients and the people who care for patients first if the administrator is not willing to do this each day, every day and every time.

Administrators must be willing to do extra work and make smart decisions. Administrators must be willing to take calculated risks and be willing to fail personally in order to make their organization successful. A great example of this is with staffing their hospitals. Many administrators hire staffing companies in order to staff their emergency department, their hospital with hospitalists, radiologists and anesthesiologists. Some are now contracting for orthopedists and others. While there are advantages to doing so and, in some cases, this may be the best solution, often this is done for convenience and because it is a "safer" solution for the administrator. Convenience because an administrator can call one company and get many staffing areas taken care of. But at what cost? The staffing company is not in the business to do favors or lose money, it contracts and charges lots of money to pay the physicians, make a healthy profit and have a cushion built in.

If administrators eliminated staffing companies, the hospital could build a more loyal staff, save money and deliver better care and service to their patients

If the administrator is willing and capable, the administrator could use multiple companies in order to get a better rate or could cut the companies out all together and negotiate directly with physicians potentially saving the hospital millions of dollars. Yes, this is a lot of work, but it is also a lot of money that could be saved and used to reduce costs to patients, used to provide other services to patients or to increase pay to those who provide care to the patients.

Hospitals keep the public in the dark

If administrators eliminated staffing companies, the hospital could build a more loyal staff, eliminate costs and have a more stable group of physicians that are happier and more likely to deliver better care and service to patients. Yet, many administrators are afraid to do this. They may not know how to do it and are not willing to learn or try to learn. Others may not do it because if the quality of care is less than desired or there are other issues, they do not want the blame. If they hire a staffing company, they can blame it on the staffing company and change staffing companies if needed. If it is done by the administrator, the administrator may be afraid they will be fired if things do not go well. So, by trying to protect themselves i.e. their job security, the administrator will allow the hospital to pay more than they must and may accept a lower quality of care. It is ironic that many administrators want employees to take ownership and accept responsibility, yet many administrators are not willing to do what they ask of employees of their organization. In addition, by not learning and being more engaged, administrators may allow staffing companies to staff with lesser trained, or qualified, personnel than might be available if they staffed directly. As already discussed, some administrators will allow staffing companies to staff using non-physicians, who are not only non-physicians and have only a small fraction of the training, but also non-physician providers that are not experienced in whatever specialty in which they are currently working and where they are treating patients. This exposes patients and the public to risks that may be avoidable if the administrators took ownership and the less convenient, possible personal job risking path.

In fairness, many administrators mean well but are duped by contract management group (CMG) representatives who have the power of CMG resources, marketing and sales teams behind them. CMGs are larger and often worth millions more than many of the hospitals that they do business with. These staffing company representatives convince administrators that the CMGs can solve problems and provide services that the hospital needs and cannot do alone. Some administrators are wise to this and do not hire CMGs but instead decide to hire their staff directly. By doing so, the hospital, physicians and patients can be much better off in the short and long run.

Chapter 8 Talking Points:

- Hospitals are notorious for being inefficient. Behind government, they may be the second most inefficient entity on the planet.
- For a hospital administrator to be successful, it helps to have certain qualities and skills. One of these is the willingness to risk failing personally as an administrator in order to make the organization successful.
- Ironically, if administrators focused less on money and more on doing what is best for patients and the people who take care of patients, many of the financial matters they worry about can get much better.
- Administrators often have access to some intelligent and resourceful people, who have innovative and brilliant ideas, that administrators often take for granted or ignore.
- Hospital administrators should leave medical decisions to medical experts.
- Hospital leaders may sometimes try to influence or push physicians and other non-physician providers to find ways not to admit Medicaid or uninsured patients to their hospital, but admit patients with private insurance to their hospital. Such behavior is not only unethical but also likely a violation of federal law i.e. Emergency Medical Treatment and Labor Act (EMTALA).

Chapter Nine:

THE PHARMACEUTICAL INDUSTRY
A.K.A. BIG PHARMA

Although drug manufacturers, collectively known as the pharmaceutical industry or "Big Pharma," typically do not deal directly with the public, they market heavily to it. It is believed the purpose of their marketing is to influence the public's attitudes and behavior. Pharmaceuticals are big business. Pharmaceutical companies make hundreds of billions of dollars every year. As of this writing, numerous pharmaceutical companies are worth hundreds of billions of dollars individually and collectively worth trillions. Based on company annual reports and stock exchange information as reported by Global Data Intelligence Center, the total market capitalization of pharmaceutical companies exceeded $2.5 trillion as of June 30, 2018. The value of the pharmaceutical companies just in North America was $1.551 trillion.[53] Profits are good too. According to Forbes, estimated profit margins in 2015 for the healthcare technology industry was 21%, making it the most profitable industry of all. One, Gilead Sciences, had a profit margin over 50%.[54]

To get an idea of how lucrative successful drugs can be, based on a 2017 Consumer Reports article, here is a list of the ten top selling medications, the annual revenue generated by each in a single year and the charge to the patient:[55]

Table 2:

Medication	Company	Annual Revenue	Charge

			To Patient
Humira	AbbVie	$13,600,000,000	$49,752-$58,044/yr.
Harvoni	Gilead	$10,000,000,000	$113,400-226,800/yr.
Enbrel	Amgen	$7,400,000,000	$49,762-$62,202/yr.
Lantus	Sanofi-Aventis	$5,700,000,000	Approx. $75 per pen
Remicade	J&J	$5,300,000,000	$39,223/yr.
Januvia	Merck	$4,800,000,000	$8-$15/pill
Advair Diskus	Glaxo Smith Kline	$4,700,000,000	$230-$370/inhaler
Lyrica	Pfizer	$4,400,000,000	$500 for 60 tablets
Crestor	Pfizer	$4,200,000,000	$170 for 30 tablets
Neulasta	Amgen	$4,200,000,000	$23,590 per year

Legend:

J&J   Johnson & Johnson

*Amounts cited are approximate

Table 2 shows ten different medications, each that generate revenues of over $4,000,000,000.00 a year. Some mediations cost tens of thousands of dollars per year, with one over $100,000 a year. This exceeds the entire annual income for many households, putting a significant financial burden on families paying for necessary medications. Some may downplay the high cost because they assume the health insurers covers most, or all, of the costs. Even if this is the case, we must be realistic and understand that the patient and public ultimately pays for the costs. The patient and society pay through higher insurance premiums. The saying, nothing is free applies. Even if insurance companies negotiate a lower cost, these drugs cost a lot, to the tune of tens of billions of dollars a year and this is only for ten drugs.

20-30% of medication prescriptions are never filled

There are thousands of other approved and experimental medications[56] and many of them are also expensive. What do the insurance companies do when they are forced to pay for expensive drugs? They raise the cost of insurance through higher premiums and justify it by arguing the high costs of providing healthcare. As discussed in Chapter 2, insurers may make even more profits since the 80/20 or 85/15 MLR went into effect. Absolute profits of the insurers can increase if the cost of medical care increases. Pharmaceutical companies and drug prices are out of control. This is part of the reason why health insurance costs are expensive. There will be those who try to justify these costs for many reasons, and we can have those discussions, but the fact of the matter is the costs of medications are too high for many patients and something needs to be done.

Zolgensma costs over $2,000,000 for a single dose

The medications cited in Table 2 are the highest revenue medications but are far from the most expensive. According to a May 24, 2019 article, the FDA recently approved a drug called Zolgensma, sold by Novartis. Zolgensma treats a rare disorder in young children called spinal muscular atrophy and costs $2,125,000 for a single dose.[57] Fortunately, it seems effective and requires only a single treatment.

There is another US approved drug for the same disorder called Spinraza made by Biogen but is not a one-time treatment. The charge for this medication is $750,000.00 for the first year and then $350,000.00 annually.[58] That is over $4,000,000.00 for a decade of treatment.

One might argue that price is not important, or should not be an issue, when it comes to your health. What parent will disagree if it means the difference between life and death of their child or loved one? The reality is price matters, especially from a population health perspective. If people cannot afford the medication or must choose between medications and feeding their family or paying the mortgage on their home, the medication's price certainly matters. People will not be able to afford them, will not fill them and thus will not benefit from them. An article published on the American Academy of Family Physician (AAFP) website reports that nearly a third of all initial prescriptions are not filled by patients.[59] The New York Times reports 'studies have consistently shown that 20 percent to 30 percent of medication prescriptions are never filled, and that approximately 50 percent of medications for chronic disease are not taken as prescribed.'[60] Another article reports that "forty-five percent of people under age 65 who don't have insurance coverage for prescriptions said they had not filled a prescription in the last year because of the cost."[61]

Whether or not you feel pharmaceutical companies' marketing of pharmaceuticals directly to the public through electronic or printed media should be allowed or is useful to you really seems moot; it occurs frequently. The pharmaceutical industry heavily advertises their drugs directly to the public. Direct to consumer advertising influences consumer choices.[62] According to a May 16, 2018 MarketReseach.com article, consumer attitudes are one of the biggest factors affecting market size, hence potential revenue.[63] If one pays attention, there are plenty of pharmaceutical commercials on television advertising various medications. According to the July 31, 2016 Motley Fool article "12 Big Pharma Stats That Will Blow You Away," Nielson estimated that $5.2

billion was spent on prescription drug advertising in 2015 alone.[64] Pfizer is reported to have spent $328 million on commercials to promote its Lyrica drug while AbbVie spent $357 million on TV commercials promoting Humira.[65]

Americans pay up to 20 times more than people in other countries pay for the same medications

What these "commercials" highlight are the benefits of the company's drug. What it does not highlight and often does not mention is the retail cost of the drug. The commercial may hint at it or mention vague statements, such as "covered by most plans" or that the manufacturer may be able to help those who cannot afford their drug but it does not state the full price of the drug. The ads may suggest or tell the viewer to ask their doctor about drug XYZ to see if it is right for them. The very fact that so many advertisements are aired would seem consistent with the claim that direct to consumer ads are effective. Otherwise, why would the pharmaceutical companies that make and market these medications, spend the billions of dollars they do on advertisement? By not discussing the full price, the public is kept in the dark thus harming the consumer's ability to make better informed decisions. Is this an oversight or is this intentional? After realizing how much medications cost patients and society and the amount of revenue that could be at risk should consumer's choices and prescribing patterns change, one might wonder if the omission in the advertisements is intentional.

Why do medications cost so much? Do medications have to cost so much? Based on findings in the 2018 article, "US Drug Prices vs. The World," people in the United States pay over double what people in other countries pay for the same drugs.[66] Patients in other developed countries pay only a fraction of what Americans do. Table 3 lists various developed countries by name and the percentage of the savings for medications as compared to people in the United States:[67]

Table 3:

Country	Average % Saved Outside the United States
Australia	60%
Canada	65%
England / United Kingdom	57%
France	67%
Germany	51%
Italy	53%
Japan	43%
Spain	55%

As one can observe from the Table 3, the same drugs can be purchased much cheaper in other developed countries than in the United States. The discrepancy can be even more pronounced in other countries. The drugwatch.com website lists some price comparisons for some commonly prescribed medications and their respective prices in various countries. We are including some of these medications in the Table 4 with the costs of either a single dose or a one-month supply (depending on the medication) and the potential savings, listed in parenthesis below the price, of the same medications listed:[68]

Table 4:

Medication	U.S.A.	Canada	U.K./AUS NZ	India	Turkey

Abilify 5mg	$34.51	$4.65 (87%)	$6.23 (82%)	N/A	$2.25 (93%)
Advair 250mcg/ 50mcg	$1,277	$377.62 (70%)	$217.41 (83%)	$84.99 (93%)	$102 (92%)
Celebrex 200mg	$13.72	$1.91 (86%)	$1.05 (92%)	N/A	N/A
Cialis 5mg	$12.13	$4.44 (63%)	$4.36	N/A	$3.52 (71%)
Crestor 10mg	$11.37	$2.04 (82%)	$1.82 (84%)	$0.39 (97%)	$0.40 (96%)
Januvia 100mg	$14.88	$4.35 (71%)	$3.04 (80%)	$2.00 (87%)	$1.17 (92%)
Nasonex 50mcg	$648	$132.53 (80%)	$113.92 (82%)	$50.00 (92%)	$43.97 (93%)
Nexium 40mg	$7.78	$3.37 (57%)	$2.21 (72%)	$0.35 (96%)	$0.36 (95%)
Viagra 100mg	$58.72	$10.77 (82%)	$8.31 (86%)	$4.44 (92%)	$9.27 (84%)
Xarelto 20mg	$15.38	$6.19 (60%)	$6.22 (60%)	$3.83 (75%)	N/A

Legend:

(%) = percentage of savings as compared to the price in the United States

U.K. is abbreviation for United Kingdom

AUS is abbreviation for Australia

NZ is abbreviation for New Zealand

*Based on drugwatch.com website, data extracted on June 25, 2018

As you can see from Table 4, Americans pay 5, 10, even 20 times more than people in other countries pay for the same medications. There are many reasons you might hear that could explain why pharmaceutical companies charge so much more in the United States. Ultimately, it is because they can. Unlike some countries, there are no policies in the United States, including price controls that limit profitability of the pharmaceutical companies.[69] Medicare, a huge purchaser of drugs, is prohibited by law from negotiating drug prices directly with pharmaceutical companies.[70] Pharmaceutical companies will argue that research and development is high, and these costs need to be recovered and justify the high prices of drugs. Some say drug prices in the United States average between 2-6 times more than in other countries.[71] As you can see from the discrepancies between prices in the United States and other countries, it appears that the United States is subsidizing drug prices for the rest of the world. Of the over $1 trillion in annual global revenue of pharmaceuticals, the United States and Canada spend close to half of the total yet only make up about 7% of the world's population.[72]

The way pharmaceutical companies, pharmacy benefit managers and pharmacies have agreements, work their pricing structure, work their rebates and do not share or openly disclose information in the easiest or simplest way to understand seems contrary to what is best for the public. There are large price differences between patented brand name medications and their generic substitutes.[73] There is also quite a range of price differences between the same generic medications. According to medicinenet.com:

"Generic drugs are copies of brand name drugs that have the same dosage, intended use, effects, side effects, route of administration, risks, safety, and strength as the original drug. In other words, their pharmacological effects are exactly the same as those of their brand-name counterparts."[74]

From the definition above, it would seem unwise to pay more for brand name drugs if there is a legitimate generic drug from a reliable and legitimate drug manufacturer. Why does drug pricing have to be so confusing to the public? Why can't they simply offer a price and stick to it? Why must they have such a high price, which they do not advertise, then discount it in varying amount, to various entities and in many confusing and complicated ways? This just seems like they are hiding something. Why not say the price is X? Because drug pricing is not done in a simple and easy to understand way, it has the appearance of inappropriateness or being discriminatory i.e. selling the exact same product in the same exact quantity at a different price to different people. The company Good RX and its website, GoodRX.com, has shed a lot of light on drug pricing and how the same medication is sold for so many different prices depending on where you buy it. GoodRX.com is easy to use website and a helpful resource that consumers can use to compare drug prices. The consumer can search generic and brand name drugs and then compare prices between brand names and generic drugs and compare prices of the same brand name drug or same generic drug prices between the various retail pharmacies in their area. Another advantage to GoodRX.com is that it is free to use and does not require the user to provide their name or any identifying information to use. The user can remain anonymous. I encourage you to visit the GoodRX website and enter in various medications you, friends or family, may be taking and see the various prices that various pharmacies charge and the discounted prices that may be available at different retail pharmacies in your area. You might be surprised at the variation in pricing for the same exact medication between pharmacies in the same town. People may realize that paying the cash price costs less than what they would pay using their insurance and only paying their co-pay.

To demonstrate the variation in pricing between Brand name drugs and generic drugs, I have chosen just a few and used the GoodRX.com website to extract the pricing information at various pharmacy chains and are including some of these in Table 5. The prices were obtained from the website on July 7, 2019.[75]

Table 5:

Brand Name Pharmacy Price	Chemical Name (Dosage/Quantity)	Generic Substitute Pharmacy Price
Wellbutrin $2101.00-CVS	**Buproprion** (300mg/30 tabs)	**Buproprion** $1768.29 CVS $37.00-Costco
Prozac $505.48-CVS $500.64-WG $500.33-WM	**Fluoxetine** (20mg/30 tabs)	**Fluoxetine** $26.00 retail-CVS $29.00 retail-WG $4 retail-WM
Cleocin $590.07 WG $591.00 WM $595.43 CVS	**Clindamycin** (300mg/30 caps)	**Clindamycin** $30 member WG $24.44 WFC-WM $90 retail CVS $27.55 WFC-CVS
Lopressor $86.07 CVS	**Metoprolol** (50mg/30 tabs)	**Metoprolol** $12 retail CVS

$83.26 Costco $86.07 WG		$5.21 WFC-Costco $14 retail WG $10.28 WFC-WG
Crestor $174.55 CVS $174.55 WG $174.53 WM	**Rosuvastatin** (20mg/30 tabs)	**Rosuvastatin** $19 WFC-CVS $34 retail WG $225 retail WM $13.42 WFC-WM
Abilify $941.21 CVS $944 WG $939.97 WM	**Aripiprazole** (5mg/30 tabs)	**Aripiprazole** $147-CVS $233.69 WFC-WG $666 retail WM $30.88 w/dis. WM
Zestoretic $426.32 CVS $421.92 WG $421.89 WM	**Lisinopril/HCTZ** (20mg/12.5mg)	**Lisinopril/HCTZ** $19-retail CVS $8.33 WFC-CVS $23 retail-WG $5.72 WFC-WG $4.25 WM

<u>Legend:</u>

Caps-capsules

HCTZ-hydrochlorothiazide

LSPL-lisinopril
MFR-manufacturer / pharmaceutical co.
Tabs-tablets
WFC-with free coupon
WG-Walgreens
WM-Walmart
w/dis-with discount

As one case see from Table 5, there can be enormous savings if one substitutes generic medications for brand names. There is also considerable variation of generic medication pricing depending on which retail pharmacy one chooses to use. Factors not well explained or covered in the pharmaceutical industry's television advertisements are the side effects or potential complications or damage that the drug itself can cause. Yes, the commercials may mention it quickly or include small "fine print" that is hard, or nearly impossible, to read in the short time they appear on the commercial, unless one pauses the commercial and gets close to a big screen TV. It is understandable from a sales perspective why this is done. They are trying to sell something to the public. If they highlighted all the harmful effects and focused on these, the consumer may choose not to ask their physician to prescribe the medication. One could say the same thing about price. If the drug advertisements disclosed the retail prices, many people would realize how expensive these drugs are and not consider taking them. Perhaps this is the point of those who oppose drug advertisement. For something so important that could benefit or harm a person's health and that cannot be properly explained to the public in a brief commercial, are these commercials beneficial or harmful to the public? Does it make healthcare better or worse? If you ever looked at the PDR-physicians' desk reference which is a reference book used by physicians to look up medications, their effects, side-effects, indications, dosages, etc., you would see the many potential side effects and harmful effects of many drugs that would scare you. But rarely do people ever read or fully understand these risks. This is potentially dangerous to the health and welfare of the public. If people do not know, how can they make well-informed decision? They cannot.

The pharmaceutical industry keeps the public in the dark

Perhaps there should be regulations requiring big pharma to not only disclose the prices of whatever they are advertising but also provide the names of 3 other drugs that can be used to treat the same condition or illness. To go further, Big Pharma could be required to educate the public as part of any drug advertisement. For example, the names of 3 of the most-commonly prescribed medications, along with the prices of each, and the names and prices of the 3 least expensive medications that can be used to treat the same condition or illness. Legislators could write and pass legislation and call it the "Drug Choice Act (DCA)," "Drug Pricing Act (DCA)," "Drug Information Act (DIA)" or whatever name they choose. By requiring the drug companies to educate the public of its options, the public would be made aware of options that it might not be aware and be better able to make better informed decisions.

Of course, big pharma would likely push back and not want to inform the consumer of other products that compete with their drug. Why would a company advertise and mention a competitor if it could help its competitor and hurt its own sales? They would not unless they are required to do so. That is the point. If the medication the drug company is advertising is so good, then big pharma should be less opposed to informing people of their options so they can make better informed decisions. If the drug is so good and priced fairly, it should do well. If the only way to sell something is by keeping people naïve or uninformed about their options, this does not seem to be in the public's best interest. Inform people and let the free market work. If everyone has accurate and enough information and the drug is the best option for the patient, then that drug should have the best chance of being chosen by the consumer and their physician. And this should be the goal of the pharmaceutical industry.

The pharmaceutical industry keeps physicians in the dark

The pharmaceutical industry does not only keep patients in the dark but also does a good job of keeping physicians in the dark. During my training as a resident, I was not always the most popular resident with pharmaceutical representatives. Why? I believe it is related to me challenging them and asking lots of questions. I grew up relatively poor. I did not have a lot of money and often went without. We were not able to afford the name brand shoes or clothes. My family had to make choices on what was needed the most. We realized that by buying one thing often meant doing without something else. I learned the value of a dollar and how difficult it is to earn money. I learned to ask questions, compare prices of things and compare the value of various items in order to determine what the best value was to me. Before I spent the scarce money that I may have had, I wanted to make sure I was making the best informed-decision I could. Many patients I treat are in similar situations in which I grew up. I can relate to them wanting to understand their choices. I asked questions so I could better understand so I would be able to help inform and better educate patients so they could make better informed decision. They sometimes had to choose between filling a prescription, or buying groceries. When I would ask questions of the pharmaceutical representatives about the cost of a medication that he or she was peddling, or the effectiveness of the new drug compared with the current less expensive medications, they seemed surprised, upset or put off. They did not seem to understand or could not relate to patients having to choose between medications and food. They did not seem to understand why I would care how much medications cost. They seemed to expect me, and the other resident physicians, to not question them and prescribe the drug they were trying to sell.

During my training and the first part of my medical career,

pharmaceutical company and medical device maker reps were known to come into hospitals and "sponsor" lunches or evenings out for the residents. While a resident physician at a busy teaching hospital, it was common for pharmaceutical and medical device maker reps to ask to take resident physicians out for drinks or dinner. They often would sponsor a lunch, dinner, a journal club, golf outing or other event. This was an opportunity for drug company representatives to "educate" prescribers about a medication or other product that their employer manufactured, distributed or sold. Most resident physicians attended for the free food. I attended many "free lunches" that pharma sponsored for our emergency residency program's journal clubs and morning conferences, and many others for other residency programs that fellow resident friends of mine invited me to i.e. orthopedics, internal medicine, general surgery, pediatrics, cardiology, neurosurgery, etc. Resident physicians liked it because as a resident, you work a lot of hours and are not paid very much, and like most everyone else, enjoy being treated to a nice lunch, dinner or drinks on occasion. As an aside, I calculated my hourly pay for the first week of my internship, that I had worked 111 hours, and discovered that I grossed less than five dollars ($5) per hour for the week before taxes. In case you are wondering...there are a total of 168 hours in a week.

Nothing is Free-Ultimately the patient will often pay for more expensive medications through higher insurance premiums, co-pays, etc.

One example is Bextra, a new non-steroidal anti-inflammatory drug (NSAID) made by Pfizer used to treat arthritis, that was being peddled by the pharmaceutical representative during the first part of my career. Celebrex, another NSAID made by Pfizer, and Vioxx, a NSAID made by Merck are other examples of drugs used to treat certain conditions i.e. arthritis and complaints i.e. joint and back pain that "old" time proven inexpensive medications such as ibuprofen are used to treat. At the time, I asked the rep about the cost. Typical answers were that they were not sure, about the same as other anti-inflammatories, or that no cost to insured patients, as it was covered under insurance plans. They would often add that it was better because it required less frequent dosing i.e. once a day, rather than every 6 or 8 hours. Their point being that the patient would be more likely to be compliant since the patient only had to remember to take the medication once a day. When I asked how it was better, the rep would sometimes produce a paper showing a research study that was done. If one read the paper, as an obsessive-compulsive resident or young physician sometimes does, one would see the official looking paper was a study that was often done by a researcher or reviewer who was paid by the pharmaceutical company that made or distributed the drug; the papers and research were biased. This is a big red flag in the science and research world that tries to minimize and eliminate research bias. Even the papers produced by these biased parties would often show little to no difference in outcomes that met statistical significance. Basically, the medication that the rep wanted me to prescribe to patients with arthritis and musculoskeletal pain i.e. joints, muscles, etc., cost several dollars per tablet. Compared to ibuprofen which is an anti-inflammatory that costs a few cents a pill, it was hundreds of times more expensive and really did not work all that much better, if at all. The inexpensive drugs also had withstood the test of time and we have had time to know more about the potential risks and benefits from experience as compared to a new and unfamiliar drug. A few dollars a pill may not sound like that much for a prescription medication but when one considers these medications are taken for long periods of time, sometimes indefinitely, the extra cost could be in the thousands of dollars. That is a lot of money. Even if the insurance company did pay for it, which I am not sure they did, what do you think the insurance company will likely do? They would likely raise the cost of the health insurance premium to make up for the extra costs of providing the higher costs of drugs and care. As I mentioned before, nothing is "free." Ultimately, the patient will often pay for the more expensive medications through higher insurance premiums, co-pays, etc. To make things worse, it turns out that some of these anti-inflammatory medications were later thought to cause harm. Pfizer was asked by the Federal Drug Administration (FDA) to remove Bextra from the market because of risks of heart, skin and gastrointestinal problems i.e. stomach problems. Specific warnings were required to be placed on Celebrex out of concern for increased risk of heart attacks and strokes.[76]

Many physicians are not as inquisitive as me. They take the drug rep at their word. Perhaps they are too trusting or did not to want to be rude or rock the boat. Perhaps they were young and naïve. Maybe they were polite, shy or embarrassed to ask or challenge the reps. Maybe they did not want to risk not getting the perks? Maybe the residents were simply too tired from the long hours to think clearly. Maybe it was one of these, none of these or a combination of these. Whatever the reason, they often wrote for the new medicine that the "nice" pharmaceutical rep represented and told us about. As a result, the pharmaceutical company made lots of sales. I was a little reluctant to change the way I practiced without sound reasoning, so I continued to use the less expensive, effective and time-tested generic drugs such as ibuprofen. By not doing so, I became less popular with the reps than when we first met. I am convinced that pharmaceutical companies have a way to track how many prescriptions each doctor writes. With time, drug reps who once seemed very interested in talking with me, seemed less and less interested and more interested in talking with residents who prescribed the medications that the rep sold.

As mentioned, the pharmaceutical companies liked sponsoring lunches and dinners to the resident and attending physicians because it was a relatively low cost to them and it allowed them time with people who are responsible for determining what medications to use or prescribe to their patients. They knew that doctors are the ones that order medications or choose what medical device to use. If the pharmaceutical rep could persuade doctors that their medication is "better" or easier to prescribe, they can easily recover the costs of the lunch or dinner for numerous physicians with only a few prescriptions. Furthermore, they know each physician often writes dozens of prescriptions each week. The return on their investment (ROI) for the pharmaceutical company is quite good. The ROI may even be better for device makers. If the medical device maker rep can convince the surgical resident or attending physician that the medical device was better, easier to use or required less effort from the surgeon, the medical device maker could make thousands of dollars from a single surgery i.e. hip replacement, pacemaker, etc. It was not uncommon for residents and attending physicians to do multiple surgeries in a single day. If representatives of pharmaceutical companies and medical device makers could influence the choices of doctors, especially the younger residents still in their training, big pharma and device makers would financially benefit for decades to come. These physicians will write tens of thousands of prescriptions and do thousands of surgeries during their careers and I am just referring to the doctors at one teaching facility in one city. This practice of "courting" resident physicians by big pharma occurred across the nation.

I really don't think the doctors knew how much these medicines cost compared to others that were as effective. Perhaps if they did, their prescribing patterns may have been different. The point is that even though physicians are typically intelligent and more educated than the average person, they too are kept in the dark by the pharmaceutical industry about pricing of medications. Drug companies don't just keep the public in the dark. Big pharma is effective at influencing many physicians' behavior and how they practice. This has the potential to be good but can also be very dangerous. Big pharma spends an enormous amount of money and by doing so, has the potential to influence physicians, especially those who want to be liked by pharmaceutical reps or who may not question the information big pharma reps "feed" them. Sometimes the influence can be obvious while other times it can be subtle, and the doctor may not even be aware of their own bias that may stem from big pharma's efforts of marketing, advertising, funding, and influence. I believe that most physicians really do mean well and want what is best for patients. I also believe that if physicians are better informed, they will make better decisions. A great example of this occurred when I served as the chairman of the department of emergency medicine and medical director of two emergency departments of a hospital organization.

Sometimes the expensive drug does not work and the cheap one does

The hospital was having financial issues and looking for ways to try to minimize losses and looking for ways to reduce costs. An area identified as an opportunity to save was in the selection of medications ordered by physicians within the hospital, specifically intravenous (IV) medications, and specifically IV antibiotics ordered in the ER and inpatient settings. As part of my duties, I attended many meetings and heard administrators complain and express their concerns. There was consideration of restricting what medications doctors would be allowed to order. Physicians attending the meetings, expressed their concern that physicians should be the ones to determine what medication is most appropriate for the patient. I understood the views of both sides. I agree that physicians are best qualified to determine the best medical treatment for patients. Of course, I am biased being a physician, but over the years have realized that no one seems to be a better advocate for the patient than a good physician, often the emergency physician, but that is a whole different topic. I also understand that it is important to be cost conscious and as long as it as effective, choosing a less expensive option is usually a good thing. Just so the reader understands, there are many antibiotics used for different types of bacteria causing different types of infections. Depending on the infection, the location of the infection i.e. skin, respiratory system, etc., the suspected organism causing the infection, the patient's underlying health condition and other co-morbidities, the resistance of certain bacteria in certain locations; there is often a choice of more than one antibiotic, often numerous ones, that will work well for the same bacteria and are effective in the treatment of a patient with a particular infection. There are often many choices, sometimes there are few and in rare cases, there may be none. The most expensive medication may not be the best choice not only from a cost standpoint but also from an effectiveness, or bacteria killing, standpoint. Organisms are often resistant to the more expensive drugs yet very sensitive to much less costly drugs. This may be a result of the over-prescribing of antibiotics or frequent use of the more expensive, popular antibiotics. Bacteria can sometimes mutate and become resistant to the antibiotic's ability to kill the organism. To put in very simple terms, sometimes the expensive drug does not work and the cheap one does.

During emergency department staff meetings, we would inform the physicians of the challenges the hospital faced and their desire to try to control costs and save money to improve the hospitals financial health. It is my understanding that similar conversations were held throughout the hospital with hospitalists and other physicians to lessen the costs of treating patients with expensive antibiotics. Apparently, prescribing patterns did not significantly change, and the hospital efforts were not achieving the intended goals. We did not see much of a change in the emergency department prescribing patterns and I do not think there was much of a change for inpatient care either, at least initially or for a few months. Of course, some in the hospital blamed the problem on the emergency physicians saying that whatever IV antibiotic started in the emergency department was often continued during the entire hospital stay.

Trying not to assign blame, I looked for a solution for the hospital's challenge. Being the inquisitive medical director of the emergency department, I called the hospital pharmacy and asked the pharmacist to provide me the costs to the patient and to the hospital of some of the most commonly prescribed antibiotics, both IV and oral, used in the ER. The pharmacist supplied me the list of antibiotics and the cost to the patient for each. The costs and charges varied considerably between the various antibiotics often used for the same type of infections.

I made a few assumptions:

- Physicians are reasonable people and want what is best for their patients.
- Doctors do not like to be lectured to or told how to practice medicine, especially by administrators who are not physicians nor have the medical training, medical understanding or that special doctor-patient relationship with patients, as they do.
- Physicians wanted to do the right thing for their patients.

I developed a plan based on these assumptions and the information I learned and did a simple thing. Without lecturing anyone or "pushing" anyone to do anything about costs, prescribing patterns, hospital challenges or instructing the physicians to do anything other than what was best for their patients, I posted an orange colored, letter-sized piece of paper with the names of the most commonly ordered antibiotics, along with the price of each, and posted the price sheets in the doctors' and the non-physician providers' work areas. Within one month, we saw changes in the ordering patterns of physicians when antibiotics were ordered in the emergency department and within the hospital. The results were great. The patients received proper care and treatments, the costs to the patient and the hospital were reduced, the physicians maintained their independence and freedom to determine what was best for their patients and the administrators were happy that costs were reduced. The lesson of the story is that the physicians were in the dark. Yes, they had enough information to make good decisions on proper selection of antibiotics that worked on bacteria causing infections. They learned this in medical school, residency training or through continued medical education. They did not have enough information to make well-informed decisions to make proper selection of antibiotics that included costs to the patient or the hospital. When the physician and other non-physician providers were given this information that they observed on their own by seeing it posted in their work area, they chose to order the "right" antibiotic for the patient based on effectiveness and costs on their own. This is consistent with the assumption that doctors want what is best for patients and want to do the right thing. This simple example shows that by making useful information easy and convenient to access and understand, people make better informed decisions and good choices. By understanding people, making reasonable assumptions, knowing necessary information, using a little imagination and applying common sense, I was able to provide the information to the physicians and non-physician providers in a creative and simple manner that helped influence them to make better informed decisions that aligned with what they wanted with what was best for the hospital and their patients. We need to do more of this with doctors and everyone involved in healthcare.

Retail Pharmacies

Retail pharmacies could also do a better job helping to educate the public and helping people understand their options so they can make better informed decisions and choose what is better for them. Some pharmacists rush through or simply go through the motions and really do not help patients truly understand enough information about the medications they will be taking. In fairness, many pharmacists do take the time to properly explain information about medications and their risks and side effect, at least to some extent, so the patient can be better informed and better understand their illness and the possible side-effects of the medications.

In October 2018, President Donald Trump signed a bill into law that banned "gag clauses" related to pharmaceuticals

Up until 2018, many pharmacists were prohibited from telling customers about useful pricing information that could help customer save money by paying the cash price, as opposed to using their insurance plan, to buy the same prescription drug that was prescribed to them. Pharmacists were prohibited by "gag order" clauses in the contracts that pharmacies had signed with pharmacy benefit managers or pharmaceutical companies. Many pharmacists faced fines or other disciplinary action if they broke these contractual "gag orders." These "'gag order' clauses in contracts between pharmacies and insurance companies or pharmacy benefit managers-those firms that negotiate prices for employers and insurers with drugstores and drug makers"[77] were common for years.

In 2013 the cash price for 1 in 4 drugs was lower than the co-payment of insurance plans for the exact drug[78]

It was not until October 2018 when President Donald Trump signed a bill into law that banned such "gag order" clauses. The bill, prohibiting the "gagging" of pharmacists, was passed with bipartisan support. Hopefully, legislators can continue to come together and pass other, well needed and beneficial healthcare legislation that can help fix our current broken healthcare system. The law does not make it mandatory for pharmacists to tell customers, but it does prohibit anyone from prohibiting the pharmacist from informing the customer if there is a lower price option. One hopes that pharmacists will choose to inform patients of less expensive options; time will tell. According to a Kaiser Health News article, NBC news reports that in 2013 the cash price for 1 in 4 drugs was lower than the co-payment of insurance plans for the exact drug and patients overpaid more than 33% for 12 of the 20 most commonly prescribed drugs.[79]

Prior to this October 2018 law, if a pharmacist informed a Medicare or private insurance plan customer that the cost to the customer using the insurance and paying the co-pay was higher than the price a customer could pay using no insurance i.e. the cash price, the pharmacist or pharmacy could be penalized. This penalty could be in the form of a fine or being dropped from insurance networks. Who decided this was a good idea? The customer can get the same exact medication for a lower amount and the pharmacist knows this and wants to tell the customer but is not allowed to? Why would a pharmaceutical company, a pharmacy benefit manager, an insurance company or any other company intentionally write such a restriction or gag clause into a contract to keep patients in the dark? While I am a big proponent of the free market and capitalism, particularly Benevolent Capitalism (BC), I am not a fan of hiding important and useful information from the very person that the healthcare complex should be most concerned about helping, the patient. This is just one more example of how broken our current healthcare system is and how the healthcare complex keeps the public in the dark.

To the credit of many pharmacists, they realized some time ago that by trying to be helpful and trying to focus more on the customer, they earn the trust of the customer and this keeps the customer loyal to the pharmacy. Customers gain value from pharmacists' help, opinion, answering questions and taking the time to explain things and trying to be helpful. Even though the extra time may not be rewarded immediately, trust and loyalty develop over time and the customer may purchase not only their prescriptions at the pharmacy but also other items such as over the counter medications, snacks, beverages, etc. The customer may choose to shop at the pharmacy over other competitors. Whether the pharmacists provide this service voluntarily, are encouraged to do so by corporate policy or are legally required to do so, the result is this behavior aligns the best interest of the pharmacy, the pharmacist and the best interest of the patient. Even if the pharmacy company encourages this for no other reason but to maximize its profits that would be OK, the behavior helps the patient, and everyone wins. One can argue that the pharmacy should profit and deserves to because the behavior that adds profits to the pharmacy also helps the patient.

Pharmacies can make getting information easier and less embarrassing or awkward. Having a "Medication Menu" that lists every medication the pharmacy carries, and the retail price, cash price and discounted insurance price, should be available in print, like a menu of a restaurant. It could list medications in alphabetical order or by what diagnosis or condition that the medication is used to treat. This should also be available online. The retail price should be listed and if a customer has insurance and enters their insurance information, it should list the specific price for that insurance plan i.e. the total cost and the customer's portion or co-pay, along with the pharmacy's "cash price." This will allow customers to be able to easily see and compare their options and make better informed decisions i.e. choose the best option for themselves. As with other medical menus discussed, it should be patient-obsessed©. The access should be easy, simple to understand and posted in a prominent location, in a very conspicuous manner and accessible anonymously. This will help better inform the public and help people make better informed choices.

GoodRx has opened the eyes of many consumers. Using this company's website allows the user to see the cash price charged at various pharmacies and the wide variation in pricing for the same exact drug. It is my understanding that the prices shown are "cash" prices and apply when not using any insurance. The user can enter his or her location to view the pharmacies and prices in that location. It almost seems impossible that someone might pay 2, 3,4 or 10 times more for the exact medicine just because they assume the price is the same everywhere; it is not. This lack of information hurts the public, the sick, vulnerable, and especially those who can least afford the high costs of their healthcare. Shedding light on the darkness that pharmaceutical companies, hospitals, and others in healthcare cast on pricing is a great way to help consumers make better informed decisions. Educating oneself and possessing knowledge immediately helps us make better informed decisions on healthcare. As a country, we should demand transparency in healthcare pricing everywhere.

Chapter 9 Talking Points:

- The United States and Canada account for over 50% of the more than $1 Trillion spent annually worldwide on pharmaceuticals yet only make up about 7% of the world's population.
- Drug companies spent over $5 Billion on drug advertising in 2015.
- There are at least 10 drugs that generate over $4 Billion a year in revenues. The drug Humira generates over $13 Billion a year in revenue.
- There is one drug called Zolgensma sold by Novartis used to treat a rare disorder called spinal muscular atrophy that costs over $2 Million for a single dose
- The same drug may cost 10-20 times more in the United States than in other countries
- Generic drugs are essentially the same drugs as their Brand name counterparts but cost much less than the Brand name. An example is Fluoxetine, the generic for Prozac. According to GoodRX.com, the generic fluoxetine costs $4 for a prescription of thirty 20mg tablets at Walmart, while the Brand name Prozac costs over 100 times more at Walmart ($500.33) for thirty 20mg tablets

Chapter Ten:

GOVERNMENT

Government has a duty to represent the people. One would think it also has a duty to do what is best for the people they represent. Many in government attempt to do this. Unfortunately, it appears that some in government do not. They seem to be more concerned about their own careers and personal well-being than the people, states, and country, they represent. Government often creates many regulations and requirements that cause inefficiencies and that are not in the best interest of the public. They pass laws that potentially change healthcare for the worse and avoid passing legislation that could make healthcare great.

Do we really know what information is contained when we click on and "Agree to the Terms and Conditions"?

One way to help the public is to make things simple. Often, there is lots of paperwork with lots of information containing legal or medical terms that an ordinary person does not understand. There is often so much information that the information becomes "noise." There is so much to read that patients often do not read any of it. This applies to insurance policies, medication side-effects, informed consent forms and most any other forms or items intended to communicate information to the public. The disclaimers really do not serve the public in the manner for which they were designed, to inform the public and help them understand or agree to the risks. The amount of time it would take people to read and understand this information is excessive in the opinion of many. Because of the legal environment in which so many are "sue happy," not only physicians but also pharmaceutical companies, pharmacies, hospitals and others in healthcare often give so much printed or electronic information to the patient to meet regulation requirements and protect themselves from liability, that the patient ends up not being properly informed, exactly the opposite result of what is desired or intended.

If government would pass tort reform, the forms could be simpler and help people understand the basics and most important points. The consents or information page could be a single page that people would be able and more likely, to read. When someone gets five (5) or ten (10) pages of information or risks of a procedure, how many people do you think read them? Does the patient really know what is in it? Is the patient really informed? Think of all the info in a mortgage loan that people sign without reading dozens of pages of boring financial and legal terms. Think of all the terms and conditions people click on and "agree to terms and conditions" online, do we really know what information is contained in them or what the terms and conditions are? Ideally, people will read everything and will understand every detail. Realistically, most people do not read everything. Even if they did, they may not understand the terminology or what the disclosure means. If we make things short and simple, we dramatically increase the chances of people reading and understanding. Perhaps we can have the current informed consent and a "highlight consent form" that is a simple one-page simple summary. It is very unlikely this will ever happen without tort reform. Of course, for anyone interested in reading in detail, the public should be given access to printed or electronic information, of the long version with all the legalese and every detail, the public can read. In addition, consumers should always be able to ask any question they would like to help them better understand anything regarding their healthcare and there should be some mechanism where consumers can easily get answers to their questions. This will help make healthcare simpler for the public to understand, this is a good thing.

Some might argue that if the pharmaceutical companies, hospitals, pharmacies and doctors provided Medical or Medication Menus to patients to help the patient be better informed, they could be accused of colluding in order to price fix. The argument is that by publishing their pricing information, all competitors would know what everyone else is charging and thus could be used to artificially set the prices higher than might occur under ordinary free market conditions. People can argue almost anything. Of course, one could just as easily argue that by hiding pricing from the public allows people to be charged higher prices than if there were medical menus. Many people are embarrassed or feel awkward to ask about pricing. By having an environment where it is difficult for the public to easily get this important pricing information, it prevents people from making the best-informed decisions. It prevents people from shopping around for the best price and value. The current broken healthcare system sets people up to be taken advantage of and to pay much higher prices than they should or might otherwise. Another option would be for government to pass a law allowing Medical or Medication Menus, providing legal exceptions thus avoiding any anti-trust concerns.

Government plays a big role in healthcare. In addition to passing legislation that governs healthcare, government is one of the largest payers (insurers) in healthcare. Medicare, Medicaid and Tricare are all forms of government health insurance. As mentioned earlier, in 2017, the government spent $1.5 trillion on healthcare related expenses.[80] The government has agencies that establish policies and regulations that can force payers or providers to adhere to. Even private insurers, that are separate from government insurance, often follow what government does even if not required to do so. For example, a private insurer may elect to not reimburse for a procedure for which the government does not reimburse.

Government is very influential in healthcare. This can be good and bad. An entire book could be written on this topic. Instead, we will discuss how government could make changes that might improve our healthcare system. A quick and simple solution would be to give the public more options. Typically, with increased options, competition works to help drive quality higher and costs lower.

Government should pass laws that promote competition and enable insurance companies to sell nationally. As is discussed in the insurance section, the government could pass or change legislation that would allow insurers to offer policies to people across state lines. This alone would help increase options to the public and could lower the costs of health insurance. Government needs to consider having national medical licensing for physicians. This is particularly important in our society and as technology has a greater influence on medicine with things such as Telemedicine and Telehealth. National licensing would immediately increase the supply of physicians that can treat the public anywhere in the United States by removing many of the costs and barriers for physicians, including specialists that are often scarce in various areas, and allow them to offer their expertise to patients who need and would benefit from it. This would be especially helpful to those who live in areas that have poor access to necessary physician specialists.

Americans subsidize the drug Research & Development costs for people around the world

Government can do a better job negotiating better rates for goods and services. This is especially true for medications. Just as people in the United States pay more than people in other countries do for the same drugs; the United States government pays much more than for the exact same pharmaceuticals from the same vendors than governments of other countries do. It does not use its great buying power to negotiate better deals for our country and its taxpayers. One might argue that government should demand that pharmaceutical companies charge similar rates for similar medications in the United States as they do in other countries. There is an argument that the United States should get a lower price than other countries since it purchases larger quantities than other countries i.e. volume discounts. As you might recall from Chapter 8, the United States and Canada are responsible for over 50% of all drug revenues. Pharmaceutical companies argue that the high and rising costs are necessary to pay for expensive research and development (R&D). There is some truth to this. Even so, why does the United States and its citizens have to pay a disproportionately higher portion of these expensive R&D costs? Other countries only pay a fraction of what Americans pay for the same drug in their country. Put another way, Americans subsidize the drug R&D costs for people around the world.

Education

Government should encourage education of the public by everyone in healthcare. Each player in healthcare complex should be required to make sure reasonable efforts are made so the patient understands and is able to make a well-informed decision. Government should require schools to teach healthcare in schools. Given the importance of healthcare and the trillions spent each year on healthcare, there is a lot to gain by having an informed and educated population. Part of everyone's curriculum should include:

- Understanding healthy diets and unhealthy diets, healthy and unhealthy lifestyles
- Understanding health insurance policies
- How to read and interpret insurance policies and the language within those policies
- Learning there are resources of where to find information related to one's health including how to find safe medications at better prices
- Understanding what healthcare resources that are available to receive care and how to determine the most appropriate facility to go in order to receive appropriate care
- How to determine the quality of a hospital or physician

- Important questions to ask your doctor and before leaving their office or place of practice
- Important questions to ask hospital representatives before treatment and before leaving the hospital
- How to find and compare costs and quality of services of physicians, NPPs and hospitals
- Understand that people can negotiate prices with doctors, hospitals and other medical entities
- How to avoid being misled or misinformed and to verify or refute information they may be told
- How to avoid being overly influenced by direct to consumer marketing, etc.

Before graduating, students should be tested on this information to ensure they have a basic knowledge base in healthcare that will allow them to make better healthcare decisions. It will put them at a great advantage to the many, uninformed, often naive healthcare consumers in society today. It will better prepare them to be healthier, require less resources and help save government and society billions, if not trillions, of dollars in addition of all the pain and suffering that they could avoid.

Public high schools should be required to teach healthcare to all before graduation

Transparency

Government should insist upon, and perhaps even require, that all those involved in the healthcare complex be transparent and make healthcare and the costs associated with healthcare as easy as possible to understand. Some ideas to do this would be to include medical and medication menus, Price-Quality (PQ) Disclosures and Policy Weakness Disclosures (PWDs). Making healthcare understandable at a 5th grade level, as earlier suggested, is one way to be sure most of the public can easily understand it.

Let's start with the insurers and PWDs. Health insurance companies should be required to clearly state the insurance costs, what it covers and how much the patient must pay. Require insurers to educate the public, their customers, by providing examples of various scenarios that clearly, and easily explain to the customer how much the customer will be responsible to pay. The insurer should be required to provide a "worst case" scenario or "Policy Weakness Disclosure" that requires the insurer to point out the weaknesses of the policy the insurer is selling. Just as a physician or hospital must explain both the risks and benefits of a medical procedure and obtain the patient's consent prior to performing the procedure, insurers should be required to clearly explain the insurance policies and give the public disclosures of the both the good and bad aspects of the policy they are selling the public before they can sell it.

Policy Weakness Disclosures should be required from all health insurance companies

A PWD would give specific real-life examples. It will explain things such as the dollar amount the consumer will be required to pay, or responsible for, should the consumer use emergency department ("ER") services for various common complaints, see their PCP or require a common surgery or procedure. This will help present information in a form that is easier for ordinary people to understand. It will explain what co-pays, co-insurance and deductibles mean in terms of dollars and cents should the consumer have medical needs or expenses. Insurers should have to give real examples using dollar amounts to show how significant charges can be and how even insured patients can be left with large bills that the patient is responsible to pay. A list of dozens or hundreds of examples could be provided to the customer to review that includes conditions or complaints by name. It should be a simple and easy to use and understand. The list would include whether the condition or complaint is covered and the total dollar amount that the customer would be responsible to pay for each. This will help avoid much of the confusion and lack of understanding of insurance policies that the public has with policies. It would also help provide peace of mind to the public that there will not be unexpected or "surprise" medical bills. The insurer should also have to give examples when there is a high deductible, co-insurance or the insurer denies a claim because a charge is not "allowed" or not "eligible." The health insurance company should be required to explain that the patient may still be financially and legally responsible for these charges and give real life examples that caused patients and their families to be financially devastated i.e. loss of family savings, bankruptcy, and loss of home or family business. In these cases, the patient's responsibility could be in the tens or hundreds of thousands of dollars.

If the insurer fails to do so, then the insurer could be fined or held liable for expenses beyond what the actual policy provides as a penalty for failure to disclose to the public properly. It would encourage and incentivize insurers to be honest and complete when explaining a policy. This way, the public might actually understand what they are buying and choose more wisely, demand better from the insurers or determine that no insurance may actually be a better option than the expensive high deductible policies they sometimes are sold. The high deductible policies can be functionally worse than no insurance at all. Either way, it is hard to argue with having a more educated and knowledgeable public so it can make a better-informed decision.

Insurance companies could make information more available to physicians and employers as well. Employers who use an insurer might request information regarding the costs of the healthcare their employees use. Specific information regarding what charges are being charged, what is the utilization rate for various items such as in-patient visits, specialists, imaging, labs, after hours care, etc. Such information is useful and important for employers to better understand the needs of their employees. It also allows the employers to shop around to get better prices. Unfortunately, this information is not always available to employers or given to employers. It gives the appearance that insurance companies want to keep employers in the dark even about the employer's own information and data. It is reasonable that employers should get this information from insurers as part of paying for premiums, at no additional expense. If insurers do not freely share this information to the employer who is paying for the employee policies and wants to use the information to better serve the employees, then government should impose stiff fines and penalties on insurers or cancel their license to sell insurance.

Big Pharma

Pharmaceutical companies have been a big beneficiary of the fast-rising healthcare costs. In just one year, revenues exceeded $1 trillion with the top eight (8) companies achieving revenues of over $530 billion.[81] Pharmaceutical companies need to be held accountable for their part of why healthcare costs are rising so fast. Changes need to be made. Some common-sense changes can begin with government demanding pharmaceutical companies to stop overcharging Americans for drugs. We understand that R&D is expensive, and companies must recover the costs of R&D for the drugs that come to market. We also understand a reasonable profit is acceptable. But what is reasonable? Pharmaceutical companies made over $1 trillion in revenues just in North America and are reporting record profits. Compensation to CEOs and other executives is in the tens of millions of dollars annually, hundreds of times more than their employees' median income. It is no longer acceptable for Big Pharma to charge $84.99 for Advair, an asthma medication, in India but charge $1,277 for the exact medication in US.[82] The US must stop subsidizing the world. Perhaps this is part of the reason why the US spends the most on healthcare but does not have the best healthcare in the world. This should be an easy fix and government needs to make this happen. If not, then we need to hold elected officials, from both parties, accountable. Facilitate the change or the public might facilitate change in the elected lawmakers. The United States subsidizing the costs of medications for others around the world was brought to light by President Donald Trump. Like him or not, he brings up a very valid point. This is not about politics, it is about right and wrong, fair and unfair and our people's health and pocketbooks. Pharmaceutical companies seem content with the way things are, they make huge profits. Some argue that setting price controls are not good or "anti-American." There are lots of ways that can result in lower and more reasonable drug pricing without the government setting price controls.

Allow free flow of information and educate the public. One idea, mentioned in Chapter 8, is to require pharmaceutical companies to include the retail price on any advertisement. As discussed, pharma does not show the retail price of medications in their advertisements. If pharma does not like such a requirement, they can choose not to advertise to the public.

Between pharmaceutical companies, pharmaceutical benefit managers and pharmacies, it becomes a complicated mess. The public is kept in the dark from valuable price information. By keeping the public naïve, the public does not make the best-informed decisions and ends up getting hurt. Without asking whether this is intentional or not, whether it is deceitful or misleading, let's simply fix it. It should be an easy fix so long as we do what is best for the people and leave politics out of it. As for price transparency, the President attempted to force pharmaceutical companies to include pricing in advertising in 2019, however Big Pharma challenged it in court. We will have to wait to see what the courts decide.

Hospitals

Hospitals do a poor job of informing the public. Hospitals must be transparent. When one goes to the emergency room:

- Will they be seen by a physician or a non-physician?

- If a doctor sees the patient, is the doctor a specialist in emergency medicine or simply a medical doctor who happens to work in the ER?
- Does the hospital inform the public about what board certification means or the value of board certification?
- Does the doctor work for the hospital or does the hospital contract the staffing of the emergency room to a private company?
- How much will the doctor charge?
- If someone is not seen by a medical doctor i.e. nurse practitioner or physician assistant, will they know what the training and experience of that provider is compared to a residency trained board-certified emergency physician?
- If a doctor does not see and treat the patient when they are in the emergency room, does the NPP, who did see the patient, discuss the particulars of the patient's presenting complaint, exam and treatment plan with a doctor in real-time while the patient is still in the ER?
- Does a doctor later sign the chart in order to meet certain legal or billing requirements and is never really involved in the actual care in real time?
- Is the charge the same for a medical doctor without emergency medicine training as it is for an emergency specialist?
- What is the charge if you are not seen and treated by a physician?
- Do the doctors who the hospital allow to practice within the hospital accept your insurance?
- What is the quality of care of the doctor(s) who practice in the ER?
- What are the quality ratings of the other doctors who may be involved in your care? I.e. radiologists who interpret images, pathologists who oversee labs, surgeons, anesthesiologists, etc.
- Are the other physicians involved in a patient's care board certified in their respective specialties?
- Is the patient treated by these specialists or by NPPs?
- Does one know the cleanliness of the hospital?

- How likely is it for someone, who goes to the hospital for unrelated reasons, to get an infection because they were in that hospital? These are sometimes referred to as nosocomial infections.
- If one requires surgery, what is the likely outcome, recovery time and cost associated with each of the surgeons and staff involved and how does that compare with other local, state, regional, private, public and national hospitals?

While some hospitals are required to track and make some of this information available, why isn't this known and common knowledge to the public? Why shouldn't hospitals be required to tell you this before you receive services or are admitted to the hospital? One would think this information is important and would factor into the choices people make concerning their healthcare. Does the public, know where to go to find this information? Do people know who to ask about it? Why do people even have to ask? Some may feel uncomfortable asking or afraid they may be treated differently if they ask too many questions or want to know certain things, so they may not ask. Some may fear retaliation or discriminatory behavior from doctors or staff members who might be offended if the patient or consumer questions them. The information should be easily available for the public to find and know without the hospital ever knowing who looked at the information. Any member of the public should be able to remain anonymous to the hospital to eliminate any risk of retaliation or biased treatment towards them. Perhaps easy to find and clearly marked links on the website home page that contains all this information should be available for anyone to be able to view anonymously. The information should be easy to understand and in plain English and other languages when appropriate. If the patient is not fluent in English, the information should be provided in the language that the patient can understand and in a simple easy to understand manner or provide access to an interpreter. If a consumer has further questions, there should be someone designated that the public can ask. Regardless of the patient's language, the patient should be able to ask any question and have those questions answered to their satisfaction.

The information should include quality measures and pricing of hospital procedures, surgeries and services. Quality measures are things like the likelihood of poor outcomes, complications or death. These should be provided along with quality measures of other hospitals in the area and across the state and nation so the public can compare. It should also include quality measures and pricing for all who provide services within or outside the hospital. It should have a listing of all plans accepted by not only the hospital but also the physicians, or NPPs, who provide services within the hospital. Make hospitals accountable. If the insurance is not accurate, the hospital would be liable and forced to honor the lesser of the rates shown or the rates that would apply had the rates been accurate when the public searched and relied on the information. This puts the burden on the hospital vendor to make sure they are transparent and provide accurate information so patients can make better informed decisions. Make it easy and simple for the public to use. Make this a requirement of any/all hospitals and require them to do this in a uniform manner so all hospitals do it in the same manner making it easier for the public to understand on future hospital interactions, should they need care again, regardless of what city the patient lives or what hospital the patient chooses.

Hospitals should be required to provide simple, easy to understand Medical Menus

Medical menus, which show the retail price for every procedure and service, along with the patient's insurance discounted price, the cash price if the patient has no insurance or chooses not to use their insurance, and the total amount that the patient will have to pay out-of-pocket should be clearly presented to the patient in a simple, easy to understand standardized manner. "Medical menus" and "Price-Quality Disclosures" can be developed and available in every emergency department and hospital that anyone can look up and view both the costs of any service and the outcomes/quality measures of the emergency department, emergency physicians and non-physicians, hospital and hospital physicians and hospital non-physician providers. Hospitals need to be patient-obsessed©. They need to improve quality and convenience, make pricing as low as reasonably possible and as simple and easy to understand. The public should be able to enter in the name and policy of their insurance and all pricing applicable to that policy should come up. The retail and patient's price for every service and procedure, including equipment and other items necessary to provide such services, needs to be provided to the patient prior to the patient receiving the service with few exceptions i.e. emergencies where delays are likely to cause harm. Total patient out-of-pocket amounts also should be required at that time. One may argue that this would be too hard to do or unfair to the hospitals. Others may raise legality or anti-trust concerns that have already been mentioned when we discussed drug price transparency. Decades ago, some made similar arguments about the airline industry and airlines publishing their airfares. The argument was that airlines would collude about fixing prices. Instead of having to secretly agree to set a price behind closed doors, the airline executives could communicate the "targeted price" via advertisement to the public and the other airlines would price their fares the same, essentially "price fixing" the fare at a higher price than might occur in a free market.

The public is better off being informed and able to shop around for better prices

One must understand, this was a time when people had to call the airlines by phone to book fares or use an in-person travel agent. The internet was not an option. As it turned out, the public seems better off being informed and able to shop around for better prices and flight schedules. History shows that publishing the airfares helped stimulate price competition and fares have fallen considerably since that time. Perhaps hospitals publishing charges can have similar price lowering effects as with the airline industry. Also, people can make better informed decisions about travel. Why shouldn't they be able to make better informed decisions about their healthcare? If we are serious about making healthcare fair and better, we must not be part of the problem but allow the public that we are supposed to be trying to help, to be well-informed, so people can make their own better-informed decision and make better choices on their healthcare.

Patients are able to negotiate the prices of care, services, testing and procedures

The same should apply for all procedures, tests, images, medications, interpretations, etc. There should be the "retail" price and the cash price to the public. For those with insurance companies that have contracts with the hospital, the hospital would be required to make these prices easy to access and understand. This is the right and fair thing to do. Inform the public and make this information easy to access. Empower the consumer to make better informed healthcare decisions. Allow them to shop around, price, even negotiate if they like. Many patients may not realize it, but one is able to negotiate the prices of care, services, testing and procedures. Hospitals and physicians do not advertise this option, but it can be done. Especially for elective testing or procedures before they are performed. This may sound odd for medical related issues, but it is like other industries or trade. Price is determined by supply and demand. If one is aware of what others are charging, a savvy consumer can use the prices of a hospital's competitor to bargain and negotiate better rates. That is why it is so important for medical menus, price transparency and for the consumer to shop around. Hospitals have a lot of down time. Their operating rooms, equipment and services are not being used 100% of the time. The cost to perform one additional test, procedure or service is typically a fraction of the retail price they charge. This gives them a lot of room to charge less and still make a profit on that additional charge.

While not as ideal, even charges for services already received can possibly be negotiated down. The reason is that many accounts receivable often go uncollected. The longer a debt goes uncollected, the less likely the debt will ever be collected. Such debt, often called "bad debt," is sometimes turned over to collection companies or sold to others for pennies on the dollar. So, it may be possible to make an offer of 20 or 30% and have the hospital accept it as satisfying the entire bill. Caution should be taken as sometimes hospitals will ask if you can make payments. If you do so without getting a written agreement with the hospital that it will satisfy the entire debt, the hospital may simply deduct it from the total and not forgive the remainder of the debt. Interestingly, after the hospital accepts this payment without agreeing that it completely satisfies the entire debt, the status of the remainder, or balance, of the "bad debt" is changed to current, which will make the hospital less likely to accept a lower offer in the future to fully satisfy the debt that is below the total amount due. Reason is that it is no longer bad debt and thus it is more likely to be collected. One reason why a hospital might agree to accepting a lesser amount than is owed could be because the charge for the service is much higher than the hospital's actual costs. The hospital has a large built in profit margin. It is possible that the hospital could lower the price by 50% or 75% and still make money. The hospital may accept a fraction of the total as satisfying the total debt because the hospital will collect some money as opposed to nothing. The "bird in the hand" principal may be one way of rationalizing it. Another reason is that hospitals want to avoid the bad press they sometimes get from the public and other consumer advocacy groups for going after people for medical bills. This can sometimes result in bankruptcy.

Hospitals should be required to post how well, or poorly, they do in patient care as well i.e. quality measures. Hospitals should have to state how they compare to other hospitals within a 100-mile radius and nationally by easy to find and understand measures such as:

- How much does it cost to be admitted for pneumonia at Hospital X?

- How many days are you usually hospitalized for a particular diagnosis at Hospital X?
- How likely are you to die when hospitalized with pneumonia at hospital X compared to other hospitals?
- How likely are you to fall or catch another illness while you are in Hospital X for pneumonia?
- How does this compare to Hospital Y or Z in your area? At other hospitals in the state? Etc.

There should many factors for each reason a member of the public is hospitalized. There should also be a severity score that is easy for the public to understand that factors in the person's risk factors that may make the results better or worse for them. The key though is that all factors, costs, complications, etc., regarding hospitals, need to be easy for the public to access or find, understand and compare so the public can make better-informed decisions. We also need to place some of the responsibility of educating the public about hospitals on the hospitals.

For elective testing, procedures or surgeries, hospitals and other surgical centers should be required to provide to patients, or their legal guardian, a price-quality (PQ) disclosure, at least 72 hours before and no more than 30 days, before the actual elective event. PQ disclosure should be simple to understand, be in a uniform manner with all other hospitals across the country and clearly indicate what is being done, the retail price, the patient's price and the actual dollar amount that the patient will be responsible to pay. In addition, hospitals could be required to also provide price information to the patient of what the same procedure, test or surgery costs if done elsewhere i.e. state average, national average, price at other hospitals within 100-mile radius. This may incentivize hospitals to price more reasonably and should help eliminate price surprises to the patient. In addition, this disclosure should disclose quality measures in the form of a quality score, of the hospital and any surgeon, other physician or other non-physician that is likely to be involved in the care of the patient. The hospital would also supply to the patient the quality score of other hospitals within a 100-mile radius as well as average quality scores on a state, regional and national level. This price and quality score will help patients and empower them to make better-informed healthcare decisions for themselves and their loved ones.

Will hospitals like it, probably no. Will there be pushback and excuses or reasons why we should not do it, probably so. But we must make changes that will help make healthcare better, more affordable and do what is right by the patient. Healthcare and rules should not focus on what is easier for hospitals. It needs to focus on what is fair and best for the public.

Physicians and other non-physician providers

Physicians can do a better job helping the public be better informed so people can make better informed decisions when they make healthcare choices. Physicians too should have a "medical menu" for their services and related items i.e. intravenous (IV) medicines, intramuscular (IM) medicines ("shots"), pills, braces, crutches, splints, casts, walkers, wheelchair, laceration repair, office visit, etc. This menu should be available online if the physician, or physician practice, has a website. This menu should easily be available to any person who comes to the office. Another option would be that anyone who practices medicine could be required to submit a medical menu to the medical board and these could be posted on medical board website for the public to view anonymously. Of course, the medical board should also be required to make the postings on its home page that are easily recognized, simple to understand, navigate and are free of charge to the public. It would help if physicians spent more time with patients and helped them understand options and make better informed decisions. Unfortunately, informed consent, consultation and education are not appropriately rewarded in our current broken healthcare system and thus are often hurried through, overlooked, partially done or not done at all. This needs to change. Giving physicians the benefit of the doubt, it's not because they do not care. Physicians have limited time to do all that is needed and expected of them given the many regulations and requirements they must follow for charting, coding, billing, reimbursement, liability protection, etc. Often staffing companies, hospitals and other health organizations employ physicians and create staffing models that create work environments that are not conducive to physicians spending adequate time with patients. Many patients would prefer their doctor spending more time with them and the physicians want to spend more time with their patients; the "employed" or "controlled" physician model that lessens physician coverage does not result in physicians spending more time with patients. Nonetheless, doctors could do a better job informing, educating and informing patients. If they did, patients would be better informed and may make better decisions which in turn could improve their health, save money and, more importantly, preventing suffering.

Why should healthcare pricing be secretive or different from any other service or purchase?

Many patients may not realize it, but one is able to negotiate the prices of care, services, testing and procedures

Physicians, NPPs and facilities that offer healthcare i.e. surgical centers, rehab, therapy, equipment, etc. should not be immune to price transparency requirements. All should be required to post retail, insured and cash prices. As with hospitals, if there are other prices or arrangements with insurers, then these price schedules should also be disclosed for the various insurance carriers i.e. list price and various carrier pricing schedules. But for everyone and anyone, retail and cash prices should be clearly posted, easy to access by anyone and not require any type of commitment including name identification or cost, to obtain. For many, it seems awkward to have to ask what something costs. It should not be. When you go buy gas, a home, a meal, the price is clearly marked. Why should healthcare be secretive or different? Shedding light on the matter is a good thing. Information and knowledge empower the consumer to make better informed decisions which is a good thing.

As discussed in the hospital section, there should be a similar place for the public to check and verify information regarding anyone in the healthcare field. This website or "office" could be run by the medical board or a state or federal government designated agency. It must be a simple process for anyone to use and get easy to understand accurate information easily and quickly. Information would include but not limited to whether the physician or NPP is licensed or not? Are there any complaints against them, professional, billing or otherwise? It would be reasonable for physician offices and clinics to be required to post the website address, phone number and information about this resource in a conspicuous location just as hospitals and ERs are required to post signage regarding EMTALA. This would make it easy for the public to find out information regarding any licensed physician or NPP. This should help protect and inform the public and prevent getting medical care from someone who is not properly licensed and qualified. It would also allow the public the ability to see if there have been complaints that might influence their decision. By having such transparency, the public can be better informed and make better informed decisions.

Physicians can be severely penalized by insurers if they try to help patients by waiving certain fees

There has been a great deal of attention paid to "surprise billing." This is when a patient receives a bill after receiving care, paying their deductible, using their insurance and paying their co-pay to the hospital. One possible cause may be that the patient received care at an in-network hospital but received care from an out of network physician within that hospital. Because the physician is out of network, the amount the insurer pays for the physician services will not cover his or her fee and thus there is a balance left on the bill that the physician is allowed, or required, to bill. The physician then bills the balance to the patient (balanced billing). Because it may be weeks or months after the medical services are provided before the patient receives the balance billing from the out of network physician, it is sometimes referred to as "surprise billing." Often bills are sent to the insurance company and may take weeks or months to be paid. It is after the bill is paid or denied that the physician, or company acting on behalf of the physician, knows how much the insurer has paid and can calculate the balance to bill to the patient. Neither the patient nor the physician like surprise billing.

Here's something that I learned from many physicians and owners of freestanding emergency centers that many people don't know and should be outraged to learn. Insurance companies often require physicians, hospitals and others to bill the patient. Even if the physician or freestanding emergency center was willing to accept the insurance payment as complete and waive or forgive the co-pay, they could be severely penalized. I'll explain this in just a moment. When an insurer sells a consumer a policy, they put certain language within the policy that the consumer must agree to by signing. It states that there are certain fees that the patient is responsible to pay. One such fee is a co-pay. One reason why a co-pay is put into policies is that shifts some of the financial burden onto the patient and away from the insurer. By doing so, this may discourage a person from seeking medical services since it will cost the patient money i.e. the amount of the co-pay at a minimum. If this deters the patient from utilizing medical care, then the insurance company has saved having to pay anything because care was not sought or received.

Now let me explain the penalty I mentioned earlier. When a physician, hospital, urgent care center or freestanding emergency center (FEC) has an agreement with insurers to accept patients with a certain insurance, they agree to accept an agreed amount as the total payment for the service they provide to the insured. This amount is typically a lower charge than their normal, retail price. But rarely is a specific amount agreed upon. Instead, a discounted charge i.e. 80% of the customary charge is used. This may not be the exact rate but used to illustrate the point. In addition, the physician, hospital, urgent care or FEC agrees to collect or charge the patient for the patient's portion of the bill. One such charge is the co-pay. So, let's assume that a patient goes to a FEC and is seen by an emergency specialist, has testing and treatment done and is discharged. Assuming the patient has already met the deductible of her policy, has a 20% co-pay and the total FEC bill is $5,000, the total charge the FEC could collect by contract from everyone would be $4,000 (80% of the $5,000). The FEC staff is supposed to collect the 20% co-pay, $800 (20% of the $4,000), and would bill the insurer for the remaining $3,200. If the physician or FEC decided to give the patient a break and forgive her $800 portion of the bill, one would think that is kind and should not be a problem. But it can be a big problem. If the insurance company discovers that the FEC or physician waived the $800 owed by the patient, the insurer may not only not pay the $3,200 to the FEC but also may demand a refund for all other bills that they have previously paid to the FEC. Here's the justification or reasoning. The insurer might claim that they have an agreement to the discounted rate which is pay 80% of the 80% of the customary charge. The insurer might argue that the customary price is not $5,000 but instead $4,200. Since the FEC did not collect and has no intention to collect the $800 from the patient, then the "real" charge is $4,200 and not $5,000. Thus, the total charge for the service would be 80% of $4,200 which is $3,360. Of that, the insurer is only required to pay $2,688 (80% of customary charges). The insurer might argue that the insurer has overpaid the FEC for every other charge they have been charged in the past for other patients since a customary charge of $5,000 was used for calculations and not the "real" customary charge of $4,200. The insurer might demand the FEC to refund $512 for every patient that the FEC saw that was insured by that insurer. If the FEC saw 300 patients of that insurer at the same charge, by forgiving or waiving the co-pay on that one patient, it could potentially cost the FEC $153,600 ($512 X 300). So even though physicians or physician owners of FEC may be sympathetic to patients and willing to cut them a break, the insurers' rules prevent them from doing so without potentially harsh penalties. I believe this is ridiculous and should be prohibited. Physicians, FECs, hospitals or others should be allowed to charge what they like and be able to help patients without fear of penalties.

Government should prohibit insurers from penalizing anyone for trying to save patients money on their healthcare

Insurers should not be allowed to have contracts referring to percentages of customary charges. They should be required to state how much the insurer will pay the physician or hospital in a dollar amount and up to how much they will allow the physician or hospital to charge, and collect from, the patient in addition to that amount. Just as government made gag clauses in pharmacy contracts prohibiting pharmacists from telling patients of ways to pay less for the same medications, government should prohibit insurers from having language or clauses in contracts that penalize physicians, hospitals, FECs or anyone else who tries to help patients save money on their healthcare.

Contract Management Groups-CMGs

Staffing companies, or contract management groups (CMGs), have been around for decades. In recent years, more attention has been paid to them as they have attracted billions of dollars from private equity and seem to have a bigger and bigger influence on healthcare. Proponents of CMGs argue that they are good for hospitals, physicians, and patients. They state that CMGs bring expertise to staffing and can have economies of scale, often can staff hospitals when hospitals cannot do it themselves. CMGs allow physicians to concentrate on the practice of medicine and the CMGs can handle all the other administrative things associated with medicine that the CMGs have expertise in. CMGs can fight insurers for better reimbursement.

Many physicians typically do not know how much is billed or collected under his or her name or license number

Others will argue that the CMGs bring little to no value to hospitals, physicians or the public and may be detrimental to them. They will state that even in the circumstances when the CMGs bring some value, the fee or amount that they charge is excessive and more than any value that the CMG brings. Many argue that the practice of corporate medicine should not be allowed and that CMGs practice corporate medicine. The things that CMGs claim they are so good at often turn out not to be as good as they claim and CMGs are known to disappoint many hospitals, physicians, non-physicians, patients and the general public. Some argue that CMGs drive costs of healthcare up and quality down.

Depending on what side of the argument one stands, one can find good or bad. What the focus should be on is what is best for the public. Since healthcare is such an important thing, some even claiming it to be a human right, we need to make sure that it is protected. One way of doing this is to make sure that we protect the physician patient relationship. Most everyone would agree that physicians are the best qualified, along with their patients, to determine what is best for the patient. Therefore, it is reasonable to state that physicians, together with their patients, should determine the best treatment and care for the patient, not insurance companies, hospitals, pharmaceutical companies or staffing companies.

Government should protect the doctor patient relationship and not allow staffing companies to interfere with physicians' judgment of what is best for patients or influence the manner physicians practice. In addition, the physician(s) caring for groups of patients i.e. in a medical practice, emergency department, within the hospital, etc. should be the one who determines what the appropriate staffing level and numbers are and not a corporate entity as this affects patient care. Government should not allow the corporate practice of medicine. The one exception might be a company that is made up entirely of physicians who are providing the care within the medical practice the corporation owns.

This will protect patients from companies concerned about profits and controlling, or heavily influencing, the way physicians practice medicine or the manner patients receive care.

Many argue that corporations should not be allowed to participate in fee-splitting with physicians. Others argue that insurers and other payers should be required to pay the physician, who provides care, directly and not allow it to be assigned to a staffing company entity. Many may not realize that when a charge is submitted to a patient or an insurance company for the services provided by a physician or NPP, that physician or non-physician provider often has little to no idea of the amount of the charge billed or what the exact code for service is being billed under their name. In addition, when the charge is paid, the physician or NPP typically does not know how much is collected under his or her name or license number. Often a CMG is the one who does, selects or directs the billing and collection and requires physicians and NPPs to sign over (assign) their rights to these accounts. These same CMGs do not share this billing and collection charge information with the same physician who provided the services and whose name and license number are used to charge the patient or payer.

CMGs controlling the money is not good for physicians, payers or patients

For those who state that physicians should be allowed to use third parties to help them should they so choose, I would not disagree. People, physicians included, should be allowed to make their own choices, good or bad, and must live with the consequences of their choices so long as their choices do not harm others i.e. patients, and the physician has reasonable and fair choices. Remember, the government has an obligation to the public and that needs to be remembered. However, if a physician wishes to use a third party to help with billing or collections, those accounts need to still be owned by the physician. Any amounts collected under the medical license of a physician needs to be collected under the name of the physician, or entity completely controlled by that physician, and the physician should remain in control of the accounts receivable that were generated from the service the physician provided.

Currently, many staffing companies bill and collect hundreds of millions or billions of dollars in the name of physicians, under those physician license numbers, but once the money is collected, it immediately goes into accounts not owned or controlled by the physicians who provided the services that generated those revenues. These accounts are owned and controlled by CMGs or their affiliates. And because the physician is often unaware of what is being billed under their name or license number, there could be fraudulent billing under a physician's name or license number, for which the physician is or could be liable, without the physician ever knowing that the fraud is occurring. This is not right. The practice of CMGs controlling the money is not good for physicians, patients or the payers. If government passed legislation not allowing assignment of fees, billing or collection to entities not owned or controlled by the physician who generated the charges, this could help prevent fraud and harmful billing and collection practices.

Government could require staffing companies to do a better job of educating and informing physicians, hospitals and the public of pricing and charges. Whether one believes that CMGs should be eliminated or allowed is up to debate. Regardless of one's side of the argument, it is hard to argue that it would not be better for everyone to be better informed so they can make better-informed decisions. CMGs should be honest and transparent with physicians. They should be required to show all moneys billed and collected and all expenses in an easy to read and understand manner. If they do so and the physician understands them and wants to do business with the staffing company, that is fine. You have two parties who are informed and can make an informed decision. Many argue the problem is physicians do not know the numbers. The physicians do not know how much is being charged under their name, how much is being collected under their name and how much the staffing company is keeping or taking from what they make. Is this fair? Would you want to know? Some argue that if a physician is stupid enough to agree to this then too bad. Others may say that physicians have little choice as many staffing companies dominate many emergency departments and other physician practices, and if a physician wants to work in a particular hospital or area, and wishes to practice their specialty, that physician often must work for a physician staffing company.

CMGs argue that they do not release this information as it is "proprietary." One can agree or not. As far as I am aware, CMGs or no one else can bill for medical services provided by a physician unless it is under a physician's, or other NPP's, name or license number. There is a reason for this. Billing and collection information should not only be available to the physician but also required to be provided to the physician as part of any agreement to reimburse for services. The government should want the physician to know what the government is being charged and paying. In the event there is some over-billing or something inappropriate, physicians could be an extra layer of protection for the government; they may be able to identify incorrect billing since they are the ones who should be knowledgeable about what care was provided and if the charges match. This is an easy way for the government to have a "watchdog" over the CMGs or billing companies at little or no cost to the government.

Many argue that staffing companies do not provide billing, collection and cost information because if they did, physicians would realize how much the staffing company is taking away from them. Physicians would protest and demand higher pay, lower charges to patients or want to eliminate the staffing company altogether. If the CMGs bring so much value and are so good for physicians, they should have no problem providing physicians this information. In the free market, the physicians will be informed and determine what is best for them. If the CMGs are correct and are good for physicians, then the CMGs should not have to worry about physicians protesting the CMG's charges or the amount they make from the physicians. They should have nothing to hide. The CMGs could in fact get more support from physicians if the CMGs released the information to physicians and the physicians felt the CMGs provided a valuable service and charged a fair amount. The point is the information should be available to the very people who are providing the medical services, under whose medical license and name the charge is being billed and who is responsible and potentially liable for fraud if the charges are fraudulent.

Government could require CMGs to disclose more information to hospitals. Hospitals would be better off if their administrators were better informed. If hospitals understood the amount of money made by the staffing company on their contracts with the hospital, administrators could better determine if the staffing company was what is best for their hospital and patients. The administrators may realize that by doing things themselves, without outsourcing, they could realize significant savings that could be used to provide a higher level of care or a service that might currently be unaffordable. Hospitals could also see the charges the CMGs are charging the hospital's patients. This could potentially add a level of protection for patients against high charges going unchecked. If hospitals are aware of the charge amounts and the amounts CMGs are billing, and feel they are unfair or excessive, the hospital can encourage the CMGs to adjust the charges. The hospital could force CMGs to charge a fair or lower price as part of their contract with the hospital. Again, if the CMGs bring so much value to the hospitals that justify their worth, providing accurate information to the hospital should not be a big deal. If the CMGs are correct and they bring so much value, providing billing and collection information to hospital administrators should only reinforce what the CMGs claim. Administrators may feel the potential millions of dollars that they could be losing, by using staffing companies is acceptable and warranted.

Patients and the public can be hurt by staffing companies. These CMGs often remove significant amounts of money from either physicians or hospitals or both. By removing the CMGs, there could lots more money to provide care and services to the public without costing the hospital a single extra dollar or a physician having to take a pay cut. Some argue that healthcare costs tend to increase when CMGs are involved in healthcare. Emergency department charges for professional fees can increase as can charges for other out of network charges i.e. anesthesiologists, radiologists, etc. that are often staffed to hospitals by CMGs. If true, government needs to investigate why and if the higher costs are justified. If not, the value and existence of CMGs must be questioned, and measures taken to eliminate any damage caused by staffing companies.

If CMGs were fully transparent, provided information and allowed others to make better informed decisions and kept their "nose" out of the practice of medicine, many of the criticisms of corporate medicine may disappear. It is unlikely that this will happen as there is too much money to be made by staffing companies. Keeping hospital administrators, physicians and patients in the dark enables CMGs to make billions of dollars that they may otherwise not make if they were fully transparent and honest with everyone. They do not want to risk losing the billions of dollars generated every year. Government should enact and enforce laws preventing non-physicians i.e. CMGs, from practicing medicine, influencing the practice of medicine, handling the collections of any payments made for physicians' services or controlling any aspects of the practice of medicine.

Tort Reform

Tort reform is an opportunity to immediately improve the efficiency of healthcare and can improve access to patients and reduce costs. Government needs to take a serious look at tort law, especially as it relates to malpractice, and make laws that will help make healthcare great again and help the people it represents. It is unfortunate that this has not been done, on a national basis, a long time ago as it could have prevented billions, potentially trillions of dollars in unnecessary spending and tests that patients might not have needed other than for the purpose of the ordering physician or NPP practicing defensive medicine. Defensive medicine is practicing medicine not just in a manner necessary to get quality outcomes based on evidence-based medicine but ordering additional tests or performing additional procedures primarily for the purpose of having the results, or evidence, in the event there is a poor outcome at a later time. The idea is for the physician or non-physician provider to prove that his/her clinical judgment was correct even though the extra tests or procedures do not change treatment or patient outcomes.

Defensive medicine costs hundreds of billions of dollars annually and can be fixed with tort reform

An example of this might be when a patient comes in after a minor fall or bump to the head. The physician might take a thorough history of what happened, when it happened, how it happened, where it happened, the circumstances in which it happened, if there was loss of consciousness, if the patient is nauseated or has vomiting, if there is blurred vision or balance issues, if the patient is on any "blood thinners" and any other necessary or useful information. Then the physician would perform a thorough exam, including a thorough neurological exam including but not limited to testing the patient's strength in both arms and legs, sensation on both sides of the body, balance, gait (way patient walks), reflexes, eye movement, pupil size and reactivity, etc. Once the exam was completed, the physician may determine that clinically the patient is fine and can be released with proper head injury discharge instructions. Clinically, there may be no justifiable need to obtain an expensive CT scan of the head that exposes the patient to a considerable dose of radiation. This would be perfectly reasonable and would meet the "standard of care."

Because of the current litigious environment, practicing common sense and good judgment may not be enough. I previously discussed how direct to consumer advertising influences consumer behavior. Plaintiff attorneys understand this and advertises heavily. Think about all the television ads, roadside billboards, bus stop benches, telephone books, sports team schedule magnets and calendars with the names of law firms on them. "According to Oct. 31, 2016, figures from Kantar Media's Campaign Media Analysis Group, lawyers, law firms and legal-service providers spent $770,598,900 on television ads in 2016."[83] U.S. Chamber Institute for Legal Reform website projected that in 2015 lawyers would spend $892 million on television advertising alone.[84] This amount does not include what is spent on non-TV advertising. It is reasonable to assume that over $1 billion is spent annually on advertisement by lawyers, law firms and legal-service providers.

What happens if on his way to jail or while in custody, the police beat him?

Given the state of malpractice; big spending by attorneys and law firms to advertise directly to the public; frivolous lawsuits; the common belief by many, including many juries, that if anyone goes to the doctor at any point and has a bad outcome regardless of the underlying reasons for the bad outcome, that someone other than the patient is to blame, many physicians choose to do additional tests, labs studies and request consultant involvement to protect themselves from possible future lawsuits. Physicians are people too and some may start thinking and worrying. The physician truly believes that the patient is fine but starts wondering, what if the patient goes home and falls and then gets a bad head injury and has a bad outcome or even dies? Someone may say the physician missed the diagnosis. I have been told by a physician that his decision to order an expensive, and what many might say clinically unnecessary, head CT scan on a patient brought in by the police was because of his concern of being sued. The patient had a scratch on his head that occurred during an arrest. As is often the case, the patient was brought to the ER by police to get checked out before they took him to jail. The physician admitted that he did not think the history he took or the physical exam he performed justified ordering a head CT scan. When asked why he ordered the head CT, the physician said that he did not know what was going to happen to the patient after he left the ER i.e. when patient went to jail. The physician asked me, "What happens if on his way to jail or while in custody, the police beat him? What if the patient mouths off to the police and the police decide to teach him a lesson? What if another inmate, that the guy says something smart to, beats the s##! out of him?"

The physician explained that he knows the CT will be normal and not show any internal injury now and that was his point of ordering it. In case, something later happens to the patient brought in by police, the doctor can prove the patient had no injury when he saw the patient and released him into police custody. The physician said he feared a jury would be sympathetic to the patient if something bad were to happen to him. It might be assumed that it was present when the patient was seen in the ER. It would be argued that was the reason why the patient was taken to the ER. He was concerned that a jury may not know when the injury happened but might give the benefit of the doubt to the patient and find the physician liable. He added that a jury may not look at or understand the medical documentation but if there was visual evidence of a CT scan that a radiologist read as normal, then he would be safe if something happened to the patient after he left the ER. The physician told me he is happy to practice quality medicine and save costs but added that he is not going to jeopardize his financial security or the security of his family by not ordering the CT and potentially being drawn into a lawsuit for something that was not his fault or occurred after he saw a patient because he knows that a jury does not necessarily do what is fair, right or necessarily based on the "truth," it often decides based on emotions or biases.

Most Americans do not realize how much malpractice hurts them and the healthcare system

The physician did not want to be a victim of the unfair system, referring to the malpractice/legal system and the manner that it is carried out and abused. This was a very-knowledgeable, qualified and respected emergency physician. His view and opinion are shared by many physicians. Whether or not you agree with his opinion or the opinion of the many physicians who practice defensive medicine is your choice. The fact of the matter is this is how many physicians think and practice. Unless we can reassure them and address their legitimate concerns with common-sense tort reform, many tests, additional consultations for specialists' evaluations, X-rays and CT scans, procedures and other costly and clinically unnecessary tests will be ordered, resulting in much higher healthcare costs to society. Many patients will continue to be unnecessarily admitted to hospitals. "DefensiveMedicine.org cites surveys that estimate defensive medicine adds costs of up to $850 billion annually in the United States. It may contribute as much as 34% of the annual healthcare costs in the United States."[85] This additional spending does not add to better care or healthcare; it is spent to protect against potential lawsuits. That is a lot of potential savings and does not even take into consideration the avoided radiation exposure to patients, the saved time, avoided complications of testing or procedures and avoided inconveniences for people.

Most Americans do not realize how much malpractice hurts them and the healthcare system. To be clear, no one is saying that we should not hold physicians and others accountable for doing things that are obviously wrong, cause harm and result in damages. I would add that the concept of malpractice is a good one. People, physicians included, should strive to do a good job, at least to a minimum standard that is acceptable to their profession, and be held accountable if they fall short of reaching that minimum standard. If someone fails at doing something that they are supposed to do and that failure was the cause of another person suffering a loss, then the person who suffered the loss should have a claim against the person responsible for the loss. Sounds simple. Unfortunately, like many other things that start off as a good idea or with good intentions, it has become something that has been taken too far and hurts patients and society. While I am no judge, attorney or legal expert, it is my understanding that in order to prove a malpractice claim against a physician:

- One must show deviation from the standard of care i.e. does something wrong or fail to do something that ordinarily would or should be done by a qualified physician
- That harm or damage occurs to the patient
- And the harm or damage that occurs is a result of what is done or not done i.e. "causation."

Malpractice cases often seem to no longer focus on reasonableness and fairness but more to reward people who have suffered injury or damages regardless of fault or causation. It has become a means for people to pay bills or financially benefit, even when there is no fault by the party they are suing. It seems that so long as there are damages, fault and causation can somehow be "imagined," "developed" or "created." Attorneys have become creative in trying to create and prove fault that a reasonable person would never find to be the case. Put another way, physicians are penalized even if they "do no wrong" or regardless of whether their actions or inactions caused the bad outcome for the patient. It has become all about money and no longer about fairness or right and wrong. This is wrong. Not only does malpractice hurt the physician, personally, professionally and financially but also hurts society. We all pay for frivolous lawsuits and unfair verdicts of juries through higher healthcare costs, potential loss of availability of qualified physicians and other providers, potential loss of available services, potentially harmful tests and overuse of resources.

Malpractice seems no longer focused on reasonableness and fairness but more to reward people regardless of fault

I will use a simple example. A 20-year-old sustains a gunshot to the chest. Ambulance personnel arrives and finds the patient still alive but in bad shape. Patient is barely conscious, very low blood pressure and near death. Paramedics start an intravenous (IV) line, give IV fluids and transport the patient to the emergency department. Upon arrival, the emergency physician immediately examines the patient, who is now unresponsive, prepares for and inserts chest tubes into the patient's chest to evacuate blood from the patient's thorax, orders more IV fluids, emergency blood for transfusion, labs and imaging and calls the on-call thoracic surgeon to make him aware of the patient and the need for his services i.e. come in to evaluate the patient and provide his surgical expertise and treatment i.e. take the patient to the operating room. This is all done in the first few minutes after the patient's arrival in the emergency department. The patient's condition remains critical and guarded and is taken to the operating room by the thoracic surgeon who is now in the emergency department. Unfortunately, the patient dies in the operating room as the bullet has done too much damage to the heart and blood vessels that the patient could not be saved. Sad story for such a young and previously healthy young man to die. The family sues the emergency physician, the thoracic surgeon and hospital for wrongful death asking for millions of dollars.

We all pay for frivolous lawsuits and unfair verdicts of juries through higher healthcare costs and the loss of available qualified physicians

It is my understanding that the claim was the ER physician should have called the thoracic surgeon sooner and the thoracic surgeon should have saved the life of the patient. It appears the ER physician asked for a call to be placed immediately upon learning of the case and the patient's status, the thoracic surgeon came in within minutes and took the patient to the operating room where the patient died during the operation. Peer review of the case reportedly did not show any deviation from the standard of care. It is my understanding that medical experts reviewed the case and unanimously agreed that there was no deviation from the standard of care. In plain English, they felt there was no malpractice. The family still sued.

The one most responsible for the death was not sued in court for damages

The plaintiff attorney's argument was that the actions or inactions of the physicians resulted in the death of the patient. What is missing and most concerning to me is the person who shot the 20-year-old was not sued. Would not one think that he was the cause of the person's death? The one most responsible for the death, the shooter was not sued in court for damages, but the two physicians who did their jobs to try and save the young man's life who was near death when he arrived in the ER, were. Is this fair? Is this right? What about society? If these doctors decide to no longer provide their services because of the unfavorable malpractice environment and move out of state, what happens to the community when there are no longer specialists to care for the injured or the trauma center closes? What happens to patients requiring emergency surgery? Future patients suffer from frivolous lawsuits. Trauma centers and emergency departments could close. The best qualified physicians may no longer be available to the public. The costs of being treated will increase to cover the extra expenses of inflated malpractice insurance premiums, legal costs and judgments. The public may have to travel long distances for care. Other than those who sue and the attorneys who represent the parties involved, just about everyone loses with a bad malpractice environment. Tort reform can help solve this.

Most reasonable people agree this is not fair or right. But lawyers continue to sue and get large judgments in cases that you might think are ridiculous or frivolous. It is my understanding that one is supposed to be judged by a jury of one's peers. Courts allow uninformed and biased jurors to judge cases who frequently are not peers of the accused. In the case I used, the physicians were "exonerated" by their peers (a panel of medical experts) who reviewed the case and unanimously found no deviation from the standard of care. Whether or not you agree or disagree with whether this is fair is one thing, but we must realize how this affects society and healthcare. Many physicians, particularly trauma surgeons have made a conscious decision to stop providing their expert services at trauma centers. Why? Trauma patients, by nature of their injuries, often have bad outcomes. While many do well with treatment, many others die or have lifelong disabilities. With the way the legal system is and how it allows what is perceived as unfair cases to proceed to trial and get large verdicts regardless of fault, many trauma surgeons have made the decision to no longer put themselves at risk. In addition to the personal tolls it takes on a physician who has dedicated his/her life to helping people and then getting sued as a result of trying to do their best to save someone when there is a bad outcome, which is inherent to the "trauma patient" population they treat, it does not make financial sense. The risk of being sued by trauma patients is often much higher and many insurance companies will not provide malpractice coverage and the ones who will, charge very high premiums. Add to this that many trauma patients are uninsured or do not pay, it makes even less financial sense to put oneself and one's family's financial security at risk when one often doesn't get paid for the services he provides and one is the target of lawsuits. So many trauma surgeons make the logical decision to stop offering their services as trauma surgeons. Some may continue to practice surgery in a private practice and no longer take trauma surgery call or they elect to move to another state that has undertaken tort reform and has more common-sense tort laws. In either case, the community suffers as important and life-saving services are lost. An example of this occurred in Nevada. All but one trauma trained orthopedic surgeon quit serving the University Medical Center (UMC) of Las Vegas because of costly malpractice lawsuits. The malpractice issues and frivolous lawsuits drove many specialists out of the state.[86]

As a result, UMC trauma center was forced to close and no longer able to serve the approximate 1.4 million residents and hundreds of thousands of annual visitors to the city. As a result, other services such as vascular, thoracic, plastic and other surgeons were no longer available to the community.[87] Many members of the public suffered. It was not until Nevada enacted laws that the trauma center was able to reopen.[88] In a sense, one might make the argument that frivolous lawsuits not only are costly in time, money and personal stress to the accused but also costly in the sense of life and services to the community and region that the physicians, being sued, serve. In addition, the trauma centers that remain, must try to take up the void caused by the closing of other trauma centers. The remaining trauma centers are now busier. As a result of the extra load, they must see more patients and can become overloaded. This overload can result in delays in treatment and worsening outcomes for patients at the remaining trauma centers. As a result, many people who may have been saved, now may die before they can reach a trauma center. Tort reform brings some common sense and fairness back into the system and hopefully restores confidence to physicians that they will be protected and treated fairly so they will be more likely to offer their life-saving services and not feel as targets. If done, trauma centers can stay open and be closer to more people should anyone require such services. Tort reform could be the difference between having physicians and services available to save a patient's life, the life of a family member or a loved one, and death.

Tort reform can make healthcare better and be the difference between life and death

Prior to 2003, Texas had unfavorable malpractice conditions towards physicians. Many believed that it was too easy to sue, and too often frivolous cases proceeded to trial. As a result, many physicians chose to leave the state and practice elsewhere. The people of Texas suffered because of how easy malpractice claims were to make and to "prove." There was a shortage of doctors. Texas finally realized this and passed tort reform in 2003. Once passed, the number of malpractice cases dropped significantly. In 2003, there were 1,108 medical liability lawsuits filed in Dallas County alone. In 2015, the number was 134; in

2016, it was 142; and in 2017, it was 126. After the tort reform was passed, physicians came back to Texas. Between 2008 and 2017, the number of physicians in Texas grew at more than twice the rate as the state's booming population growth in that same period. This is consistent with what many say that more reasonable and fair malpractice laws end up helping the community and all people. There are now more physicians who can care for the public. States that require a higher standard of proof for malpractice, such as Texas, often benefit.

The need for tort reform applies to not only trauma centers but all types of medicine. It is not unusual for physicians to consider the malpractice climate of various states before deciding where to practice their specialty. If a state has tort reform in place, physicians are more likely to practice in that state. If the malpractice climate in a state is bad, physicians may decide to practice elsewhere. If it seems too easy to sue or judgments against physicians seem unfair, physicians may also change the way they practice. While this may sound good, it often is not. If they are practicing high quality medicine already, they still get sued. So, what do physicians do, they practice defensive medicine just as the emergency specialist did with the patient brought into the ER by police. Physicians start ordering more lab tests, X-rays, images, MRI's and other tests. They refer patients to high cost specialists instead of treating patients themselves. While to the inexperienced person, this may sound like a good thing or "better care," it often is not. Outcomes do not change but the costs go up drastically and limited resources are used up on patients who do not need them. As a result of the practicing of defensive medicine, healthcare costs go up for everyone, some cannot afford healthcare at all and others are not able to get the care they need. It is hard to know for sure, but it has been estimated that America's healthcare costs as much as 30-40% higher just because of defensive medicine.

In addition, ordering more tests may be harmful to patients. Some people are concerned about the radiation they get from a single chest

X-ray. One CT scan of the abdomen and pelvis can expose the patient to an amount of radiation, and increased risk of cancer, equivalent to about 1500-2000 chest x-rays. So, if your physician orders the CT because he/she wants to have evidence that there is nothing more serious, as opposed to simply trusting their clinical judgment based on a good history and physical exam, you get a big dose of potentially cancer causing radiation and about a $1000-$4000 higher bill. Many physicians feel comfortable in their skills but in the event that the patient condition could change, they know some attorney will be happy to sue and claim that a CT scan should have been ordered and would have shown the problem and prevented the pain or suffering of the patient even though that may not be the case. It is easy to claim anything after the fact, just like playing "Monday morning quarterback."

There are so many examples of why our legal system needs updating, particularly with tort claims. An entire book, or series of books, could be written on this topic alone. One gets the idea of how making simple common-sense tort reform, could help society and help make healthcare great again.

Telehealth

Government needs to stay current and look at what is best for the public. Government should use common sense when determining what health services, it will reimburse. A good example of this is with Telemedicine or Telehealth. Telehealth is not a new form of medicine; it is simply the vehicle that enables a patient, physician or other NPP located at one location, "home site," to receive services from a physician located in a remote or "distant site" using telecommunications in real time. It is typically audio and visual. As mentioned, government is one of the biggest payers in healthcare i.e. Medicare, Medicaid and Tricare. There are many positives and negatives to Medicare. One of the most recent flaws that come to light with the advent of technological advancements is the way Medicare reimburses, or does not reimburse, for care delivered via telehealth. Reimbursement is an important factor in determining whether things are accepted or are implemented. Whether we want to believe it or not, if government or other payers do not pay for a service or treatment, then that service or treatment is much less likely to occur. Things cost money and if one is not paid for something, it is unlikely that anyone will provide those services. Typically, if government will reimburse for something, the private sector will. It is harder for a private payer to justify denial of payment if the government pays for that same service. Telehealth is one such service.

At one point, Medicare did not reimburse for care provided via telehealth. This has started to change. Medicare does in fact now reimburse for some telehealth care such as in circumstances when a service is not otherwise available to a Medicare patient i.e. a rural Medicare patient needing a dermatologist evaluation, but the nearest dermatologist may be 100 or more miles away. Medicare will also cover patients who receive care via telehealth if the patient is located at an eligible originating or home site. According to Centers for Medicare and Medicaid Services (CMS),[89] these sites include the following:

- Physician and practitioner offices
- Hospitals
- Critical Access
- Rural Health Clinics
- Federally Qualified Health Centers (FQHCs)
- Hospital-based or CAH-based Renal Dialysis Centers (including satellites)
- Skilled Nursing Facilities (SNFs)
- Community Mental Health Centers (CMHCs)
- Renal Dialysis Facilities
- Home of beneficiaries with End-Stage Renal Disease (ESRD) getting home dialysis
- Mobile Stroke Units

While the above list is a good first step, it needs to be expanded. Care should be allowed anywhere the patient is located so long as the care meets quality standards and should be reimbursed at the same rate as care provided in-person (parity). It should not matter if care is at the doctor's office, in a patient's home or anywhere else. Reimbursement needs to be based on the care, not the location in which the care occurs.

At the time of writing, Medicare does not currently cover care provided via Telehealth if that same service is available in-person in that area i.e. urban area. For example, Medicare would not cover the costs to care for a patient in their home in a large city who required evaluation if that care is provided via telehealth. Medicare would pay for an ambulance transport from the patient's home to the emergency department, the emergency department evaluation and emergency charge of the hospital ("facility charge") and physician ("professional fee") who may not even be an emergency specialist, and the transportation back to the patient's home which could be in the thousands of dollars. Yet Medicare will not pay for an emergency specialist to evaluate and treat that same patient in the their home via telehealth even though the care and outcome would likely be as good or better for the patient, not expose the patient to avoidable infections, and would potentially save hundreds or thousands of dollars. Does this make sense? Given the advances in technology and the ability of a quality evaluation by a physician via telehealth, does it make sense to have to inconvenience the patient, transport them to another facility, possibly expose them to infections within the hospital or emergency department and elements of the weather, interrupt their routine, tie up an ambulance that might be needed for another call or life threatening condition, add to the workload of an emergency department that may already be overcrowded and cause delays to other patients when that patient could be immediately seen in the comfort of their current environment and familiar surroundings at a fraction of the cost? Of course not.

Reimbursement needs to be based on care, not the location in which the care occurs

Efficiency

While the term efficiency may seem unheard of in government, it needs to become commonplace if we want to fix our current healthcare system. Government may be the most inefficient and wasteful entity on the planet. It should not be and does not have to be. We could debate the reasoning why government is the way it is and attempt to justify its inefficiency but talking often is just that, talk. Many books could be written about government and its wastefulness and inefficiencies but again, this is for another time. Those in government may have started with good intention, but like many other things that start off for good reason and with good intentions, government has morphed into something that no longer achieves many of these good intentions and has become something that has created many new unintended and unnecessary consequences, issues or problems. This needs to be fixed and by doing so we can improve healthcare and likely make other parts of society better as well.

There has been a lot of talk about the Affordable Care Act (ACA), often referred to as "Obamacare." Many people oppose it and many people support it. Often, the support or opposition seems to be based on the political orientation of the person. This is unfortunate but recently seems to be a common occurrence. Healthcare should not political. Sickness, illness, disease and death affect both republicans and democrats, independents and libertarians. It impacts all races, sexes, religions, ages, etc.; it affects all of us and we need to come together to do what is best for the individual, one another and all of society irrespective of any demographics or political affiliation. By doing so, we all benefit.

Obamacare allowed children up to age 26 to remain on parent's policies and protected people with pre-existing conditions

Two of the most popular parts of the ACA is it allows children to remain on their parent's health policies until age 26 and prevents insurers from denying coverage to people with pre-existing conditions. Another part, not as well known, is that there is a requirement known as the 80/20 rule or the medical loss ratio (MLR). The MLR was briefly discussed at the end of Chapter 2. I will discuss it further in just a bit. The rule requires health insurers to spend at least 80% of the policy premiums they collect on medical care and quality improvement measures and the remaining amount can be used for overhead, administrative expenses and profits. The law took effect in 2011. It is believed the intention of this law was to prevent insurers from spending less on patients in order to increase profits. In fact, if insurers did not spend the required percentage on medical care and quality improvement measures, the insurer would be required to refund the difference to those who paid the premiums. As a reference, Medicare maintains a MLR of 97-98%.[90]

There are two potential flaws that come to mind. First, who verifies the insurer spends the required 80-85% on medical care or quality improvement measures? Has it ever not been met? What was done to enforce the law and was there anything to prevent or discourage the insurer from doing it again i.e. fine, penalty, canceling license to do business? If the worst thing that can happen to insurers who cheat and spend less than the required 80% of revenue on medical costs and quality improvement activities is that they will have to refund the difference and nothing else, I imagine that many of them will spend less than 80%. Why? If they do not spend the 80% and they do not get caught, they potentially drastically increase their profits. If they get caught cheating, they are no worse off financially than had they followed the rules to begin with; all they have to do is pay what they would have had to pay if they followed the rules to begin with. Thus, it seems to almost incentivize insurers to cheat unless there are penalties that are severe enough to prevent cheating.

Second, what is the definition of "Quality Improvement Activities?" This is a broad term and if interpreted the right way to benefit insurers, could potentially allow insurers to spend money on buying assets that increase the value of the insurer without directly providing medical care to or helping the insured i.e. buying real estate or buildings used to house quality improvement personnel. By requiring the insurer to spend a set percentage of the revenue, it limits the percentage of revenue that is left over that can contribute to profits. At first glance, this sounds good but if one thinks about it, the potential for abuse could result in less vigilance of insurers and higher costs of healthcare. Let me explain.

Obamacare allows insurance companies to make significantly more money when healthcare costs go up

A potential benefit of having insurers involved in healthcare is that they keep an eye on doctors, hospitals, pharmacies, pharmaceutical companies and others in healthcare and try to negotiate lower prices or prevent unnecessary tests by withholding authorization i.e. denying test. I used the term "watchdog" earlier. The idea is that by doing this, patients and payers will benefit by reducing utilization and lowering reimbursement to physicians and others who provide services in healthcare. Of course, many would say the insurance industry has failed at this job. Healthcare costs have outpaced inflation and wages. One reason could be that the insurers realize that it is in their best financial interest for prices to go up. If prices go up, the insurer can justify premium increases. So long as the price increases are for medical related costs and quality improvements and the costs stay constant for administrative costs and overhead, profits will go up. For example, if an insurer collects $1,000,000,000 in premiums and pays $800,000,000 in medical care and quality improvement activities, that leaves $200,000,000 for administrative costs, overhead and profits. Assume that administrative costs and overhead are $100,000,000, the insurer would make $100,000,000 in profits ($1,000,000,000-$800,000,000-$100,000,000). Now assume the costs of medical care (costs of hospitals, pharmaceuticals, physicians, imaging, labs, etc.) doubles. The insurer now doubles the premium amounts and will collect $2,000,000,000 in premiums and will triple its profits ($300M vs $100M). If we do the math... $2,000,000,000-$1,600,000,000-$100,000,000=$300,000,000. So, while the insurer may give lip service to complaining about doctors, hospitals and others, the ACA allows them to make more money when prices go up, even though they still pay out the required percentage. Remember the mother and child bowl of ice cream example from the Chapter 2. While the intention of the ACA may have been good, it may be one of the reasons why healthcare costs continue to go up. The ACA's MLR requirement may provide a financial disincentive for insurers to be a good watchdog and keep healthcare costs low.

Chapter 10 Talking Points:

- Government can significantly impact healthcare. It not only pays for about $1.5 Trillion in healthcare expenses, it can write and pass legislation that governs the United States' approximate $4 Trillion annual healthcare costs.
- Telemedicine and Telehealth is an effective way to provide healthcare and government should require that all payers must pay for Telehealth at the same rate as for in-person care, regardless of where the patient or physician (and non-physician provider) are located
- Insurance companies should not be able to exclude any physician from providing care to their insured via Telehealth
- Lawsuits and the threat of lawsuits cause many physicians and other non-physician providers to practice defensive medicine. Defensive medicine may add over 30% to healthcare costs. This adds up to hundreds of billions of dollars.
- If there was significant tort reform, there is the potential to save close to $1 Trillion dollars each year.
- States with unfavorable tort laws may lose specialists, have trauma centers close and risk the health and safety of the public.
- The United States government pays a lot more than governments of other countries for the exact same drugs of the same manufacturers.
- Healthcare should be taught in schools so the public will be less naïve and more likely to be able to make better informed decisions, more capable of understanding insurance policies, how to select a health care provider (physician or non-physician), negotiate better prices and know what resources are available to them.
- Government must require the players in the healthcare complex to help educate the public and provide quality information, pricing information for not only themselves but for competitors within a certain area i.e. 100 miles, the state and nationally so consumers can compare.

- Government should require any payments to physicians or hospitals be controlled by the physicians or hospitals and require any billing entity to clearly inform the doctor as to exactly how much is billed and collected under his or her name and license number i.e. itemized list.
- Government should prohibit insurers from financially penalizing doctors or hospitals who offer discounts to patients or who try to help patients save money on healthcare.

Chapter Eleven:
PEOPLE-PATIENTS-THE PUBLIC

People are not only the most important but also the single most influential part of a great healthcare system. The public must be informed and engaged. The public must also be held accountable. Its influence, decisions, behavior, lifestyle, and choices can have the greatest impact on good health and making our current broken healthcare system better. By choosing to do, or not do, business with insurance companies, hospitals and others within the healthcare complex can impact how the healthcare complex players behave and respond. People take for granted their power and influence. If people voice their opinions and concerns, push their legislators and demand change, it will result in action and facilitate change. The public has power that many try to downplay, but we are a country that is based on "for the people" and if the people of the country are determined and demand change, it can and will happen.

"Simple" things that are ordinary and taken for granted in the United States, save more lives than any doctor or antibiotic

Ironically, this opportunity to impact and influence healthcare has not been given much attention. The public's behavior and choices can do so much to make a positive impact on public health and the healthcare system. As a society, we seem to focus on healthcare when there is a problem but not so much when things seem OK. I often hear about how doctors, medications and certain procedures save lives. We seem to notice what people do for the sick and injured but ignore, or do not realize what others do, that may contribute more to the health of our population. An example is infection and antibiotics. Many believe antibiotics are the answer whenever they get ill. While antibiotics do kill certain bacteria that cause a variety of infections, reduce infections and can save lives, there are behaviors and other things we can do that prevent illness from ever occurring in the first place. People seem to ignore the less exciting or not so high- tech stuff like soap and handwashing. If everyone did simple hand washing and practiced better hygiene, many infections would never occur or ever require antibiotics or other treatments. If people used common sense and covered their mouths when they coughed and did not drink from the same bottles or glasses, many infections could be prevented. Another example is safe housing, proper diets, sanitation, indoor plumbing and garbage pick-up. These "simple," not so exciting and taken for granted things, that are routine and ordinary in the United States, save more lives than any doctor or antibiotic ever has. Ever heard of the plague, cholera or how millions, maybe even billions, around the world live without clean drinking water, proper shelter or food? If these people had clean drinking water, better sanitation and the other things we have in the United States, much of the human suffering would go away. There is so much good that can come from things that may seem unimportant, mundane, boring or taken for granted, that are incredibly important. Fortunately, in the United States and other developed countries, sanitation, clean and safe drinking water and enough food is the norm. Yet, on occasion and for some, this is not the case.

Just as these things that may not strike us as being part of good healthcare i.e. clean drinking water, proper shelter and food, the decisions and choices people make are very likely more important than anything that occurs after one becomes ill i.e. the doctor, hospitals, medications, etc. If as a society, we can make sure people have access to these important and essential services, then it is much less likely they will become sick and our overall population health will improve. These are challenges we need to address. What an individual must address is his personal choices. The things that one chooses to eat, drink, smoke, or expose oneself, one's children or family to will affect their health. It may cause them to become sick or make them more susceptible to illness or poor health. Whether we decide to do what is right or what we want, as the two sometimes conflict, may determine the state of our health and lead to a healthy life or a life full of illness and poor health. Just like garbage men hauling off garbage may prevent many illnesses and diseases from ever occurring and eliminate the need of a physician's services for the prevented sickness, many of our everyday choices determine whether we will be healthy or sick. Some argue that most health problems are related to lifestyle. Simple boring things can save millions of lives, trillions of dollars and tons of suffering:

- The diets we eat that cause cardiovascular disease
- The tobacco we smoke, dip and chew that cause cancer, heart attacks, strokes, vascular and multiple lung and respiratory diseases
- The alcohol we consume that cause hepatitis, cirrhosis, gastrointestinal bleeding, brain and testicular atrophy, affect unborn babies and cause other undesired effects
- The sedentary lifestyles we lead i.e. playing video games rather than participating in sports or exercise; sitting on the couch rather than taking a walk
- The number of sexual partners one has and deciding whether to use protection or not
- The decision to use IV or other drugs or not
- Following a physician's instructions or recommendations

All the choices that we make play a big part in our health. We, the public, play the leading role in, and most important part of, our health status and the healthcare system. Do not take this for granted. Do not allow others to influence us to make poor decisions or discount our responsibility to ourselves, our families and society to educate ourselves about our health so we can make the best-informed decisions to maximize our health.

The reality is that the public is not well informed or is misinformed. Who is to blame for this? Everyone including the public itself. As important as our health is, many do not put in the time that is necessary to learn about healthcare i.e. insurance policy, hospitals, doctors or other non-physician providers or services, diets, lifestyles, to understand it. There may be plenty of reasons for this. We may not believe it is necessary. The public may trust the insurance company to take care of them if they get sick or injured. The public cannot imagine that they pay so much and not get taken care of if care or treatment is needed. The public assumes it will never need it so doesn't worry about it. The public has enough to worry about than spending valuable time learning how healthcare works or about their insurance policy. We assume that all doctors are the same or capable of doing whatever is needed. We assume that if a doctor or hospital is licensed, then they must be good enough. We assume hospitals will look after us and make sure everyone is qualified and knows what they are doing. We may assume if a hospital allows the substitution of a NPP for a physician, then the NPP is as qualified as a physician. We assume that if someone provides services at a hospital that is in the patient's insurance in-network, everyone accepts the patient's insurance. We assume board certification, or residency training in the medical specialty, in which a physician practices, does not make a difference in the quality of care. We may not even be sure what residency training or board certification means. Do not assume. Healthcare is quite boring to many and people do not want to spend time doing boring things. But the public must take some responsibility for how bad our current healthcare system is today. The blame is for not knowing more about their health plan or the current healthcare system. People must accept blame for not being more engaged and for the poor lifestyle choices they make that contribute to poor health and bad outcomes.

People must accept responsibility, need to ask questions and not assume anything

People want to be politically correct and not dare accuse or blame the sick or afflicted of making poor choices. It seems that not enough attention has been given to the public's role in and blame for our healthcare problem. This must change. If we want things to be better, we must be honest and accept responsibility. We must respect people enough to tell them the truth. At a minimum, we need to make sure we include the public, its choices, its engagement, and its role in healthcare if we are serious about making our population healthier and improving healthcare. This is no time to be so worried about political correctness that we continue to allow our population to be unhealthy, helpless and victims.

While the public carries part of the blame, there is plenty of blame to go around. Insurance companies, hospitals, doctors, and the rest of the healthcare complex collectively contribute to the problem and carry some degree of blame. Some healthcare players are more to blame than others. But if we are being honest and really want to fix things, we must all accept responsibility and change. I have discussed the various players and how each contribute to why our current healthcare system is broken in earlier chapters. One might say that the various players within the healthcare complex hide things from, deceive or mislead the public by keeping the public in the dark, misinformed, and uninformed. By doing so, the public is not able to make the best-informed healthcare decisions. One could argue this is intentionally done, others could argue it is an innocent oversight while others might argue that misinformation, deceit or keeping the public in the dark does not exist. You be the judge.

People need to learn to ask questions and not assume anything. There should be a mechanism in which people can easily find whatever information they seek or that would help them make better informed decision. People must empower themselves with knowledge, they cannot be passive or play victim and find excuses why they do not try to do whatever they need to do to become better informed or make better informed decisions for themselves and their families. This is not to excuse or defend the healthcare complex. It is just to say that everyone, including the public, should do the right thing and whatever they can to make healthcare better. They should not be embarrassed to ask questions, shop around, negotiate rates, fees, and services, expect and if necessary, demand information. They should not wait for others to start to do the right thing before starting to do the right thing themselves. Everyone should simply start doing what they can to make healthcare better now. It is time to walk the walk and not just talk.

The biggest and most important thing for the public to do is to take responsibility for our own health. Peoples must be held accountable for making poor choices, living unhealthy lifestyles, and behaving in a manner that contributes to poor health or worsening of their health. While it is nice and convenient to have others involved in the healthcare system, there should be, and usually is, no one who will care more about your health, and the health of your family than you. People are not stupid, but their behaviors often seem to be. Despite knowing better, people continue to live unhealthy lifestyles, make poor health decisions, eat unhealthily and either take a victim mentality or a passive role in their own healthcare. People say how health is so important, yet these same people do not dedicate the time and energy that proves they value it. People spend much more time watching TV, talking on the phone, texting and surfing the internet for all kinds of things other than health. If we truly believe health is so important, we need to act like it is.

If I could rid the world of cigarettes and other tobacco products, I would save more lives and prevent more suffering than most anyone else in the history of the world

Let's start with one of my biggest pet peeves: cigarette smoking. As a physician, if I could rid the world of cigarette smoking and other tobacco products, I would save more lives and people from suffering than anyone else in the history of the world. It amazes me how something that causes, contributes to or worsens so many bad things such as cancer, heart disease, stroke, chronic obstructive pulmonary disease (COPD), asthma, allergies, respiratory illnesses to the smoker and those around them including children, etc., is something people choose to do. Tobacco use kills and causes suffering of millions of people every year and has for decades. Currently, it is hard to imagine that anyone does not know that cigarette smoking is unhealthy. Even people who smoke will admit it, yet they still light up. They will give all kinds of reasons why they smoke. It is one of my few enjoyments in life, it relaxes me, it is a habit, I like to, etc. They will tell you they plan on quitting. But so many never seem to do. They may say they are addicted and are unable to quit but decline offers to help them break their addiction.

In addition to damaging one's health and the health of those around them and the high human costs, tobacco is responsible for a lot of money changing hands. On one hand, tobacco is big business and generates lots of revenue for tobacco companies. In 2017, about ¼ of a trillion cigarettes were sold in the United States.[91] People spend billions and billions every year on cigarettes and tobacco related products. On the other hand, the costs to society are enormous. In addition to the costs associated with buying the "poison," the use of tobacco is expensive in terms of how much is spent taking care of illnesses and diseases caused or worsened by tobacco use. The Center for Disease Control (CDC) estimates that about $170 billion is spent on direct care related to tobacco use and tobacco use costs us another $156 billion in lost productivity.[92] This does not even consider the suffering that the patient, their family and loved one's experience when the negative effects and illnesses caused by tobacco occur. These include but are not limited to:

- People who have died
- Those with intractable cancer pain
- People who can't breathe or get enough air

- Those who can't walk across a room without having to stop because they have destroyed their lungs' ability to exchange carbon dioxide and oxygen and properly ventilate or oxygenate
- Those who have had strokes whose healthy lives have been stolen from them, who are no longer able to walk, talk or care for themselves and are confined to a bed and develop many of the complications associated with being bed-stricken
- Those who have had a heart attack and unable to do many activities or must make frequent visits to the emergency room for chest pain, weakness or inability to catch their breath with fear of dying on any given day
- Family members or children who have respiratory problems

The list goes on and on. If anyone has a family member or has been around someone suffering from any of these illnesses or conditions caused or worsened by tobacco, they know the stress, worrying and suffering that those around the patient go through as well. Yet knowing all this, people continue to smoke and use tobacco. People convince themselves that it will not happen to them or that they will quit before something bad happens. They believe bad things happen; they just do not happen to them. They do not believe statistics. People argue that bad diseases happen even to people who do not smoke. While this is true, people ignore the fact that smoking greatly increases one's chances of suffering from many terrible illnesses and diseases. Wake up people.

Honesty is often the greatest show of respect to another individual.

We cannot live an unhealthy lifestyle and expect to be healthy; it is that simple.

When illness or catastrophe happens to those who make bad choices and put themselves at much greater risk for contracting these illnesses and diseases, many ask why me? They want sympathy and then some become determined to change their lifestyle. Some continue to use tobacco despite being stricken with a terrible disease or illness caused by tobacco. Ironically, others who are strong enough to change their lifestyle and stop tobacco, often return to the same bad habits and lifestyle. It is quite sad the amount of control that tobacco holds over so many people. It is hard to not feel empathy for those with illnesses and diseases, even if people make bad choices that increase their chances of getting sick or dying. But we should not allow our emotions to prevent us from having honest discussions and helping to educate patients and the public in hopes of preventing further suffering. If we really love people, we need to be honest, even if it sometimes is awkward or uncomfortable to do so. Honesty is often the greatest show of respect to another individual. If we focus less on emotions and more on common sense and what is best for the patient and society in general, we will stop condoning or looking past poor choices and put incentives and disincentives in place that will encourage people to make better choices that will lead to better health for the individual and for all of us. We must accept responsibility for our choices and decisions and behave responsibly. We must educate ourselves and practice prevention. It may be hard at first, but if that is what it takes to make us healthier, people will get past the initially difficulty and come to realize it is well worth doing. By the time we are sick, we have already lost. We cannot live an unhealthy lifestyle and expect to be healthy; it is that simple. If we don't do it for ourselves, we must do it for our loved ones.

Diet

Most people will agree that there are "healthy" and "unhealthy" diets. Unfortunately, many people don't' really know what is healthy or unhealthy. People are confused by food manufacturers and distributors and the way products are marketed. Many people will admit that eating fried foods, foods high in cholesterol and fats, processed foods, lots of red meat and high calorie diets is not healthy. But what do we do? Many eat lots of fried foods, foods high in cholesterol and fats, processed foods, lots of red meat and high calorie diets. Again, we know better but choose to ignore our better judgment and make unhealthy choices. When you confront these people and ask why, you get all sorts of excuses and explanations. "I do not have time to cook, it is too expensive to eat healthy, I like the taste of it." Some people may not realize that their diet is bad. They may not realize that it is not only the calories or their weight that is important but also what they are eating. Some may say that it does not matter, they will change later, or they can go to the doctor and get a prescription for a medication to help them lose weight. Some believe that being overweight is the only problem. They are not aware of the damage that is being done internally to their blood vessels and internal organs even if their weight is acceptable to them. Perhaps they truly do not know, perhaps they do not care. Unfortunately, there are many who seem more concerned about their appearance than their health. They unfortunately equate the two when in fact they can be very different.

Common sense should tell you that if you put lots of bad things in, then bad things can and will happen. Forget about the body for a moment. Think about a traditional car with a combustion engine. If you put dirty gasoline or motor oil in your car or truck, gas that may have water in it or other contaminates, motor oil that has metal shavings in it or be too thin or too thick, or if someone pours sugar into your gas tank, what happens? Your vehicle does not run well. In fact, it may not run at all and may require very expensive repair. So why do you think you can put bad things into your body and not expect bad outcomes? Yet, as humans we do this every single day.

Unrealistic expectations

People seem to have the opinion that there is an easy fix for everything. If they are overweight, there should be a pill to help lose weight or suppress their appetite. Others choose to undergo bariatric surgery in order to control their weight. If they have diabetes, that is often brought on or worsened by obesity, they expect a pill. Congestive heart failure? There is a pill for it. High blood pressure? Another pill. Wake up people. Look, we must be honest. Honest with ourselves and with each other. Instead of being offended when someone is honest and calls things as they are, we must understand it is true, not take offense but understand the facts and do things that are healthy and beneficial to us. While medications are often needed for various conditions, they should never be the first or primary thing we do to correct unhealthy lifestyles or poor choices. We need to try and live healthier, make better choices and try to prevent the condition in the first place. People do not seem to be too interested in changing their behavior. They want to eat what they want, do what they want and live how they want even if they know it is unhealthy. People want and expect a quick fix to allow them to continue their unhealthy lifestyle and poor choices instead of making better choices and changing to a healthy lifestyle that may negate the need for medications. Have we have lost our willpower? Have we become so spoiled that we expect everything to come easy? If we are obese or even just a little overweight, why not address the cause? Why not try to prevent the condition to begin with? Why not decrease our intake, choose a better diet, start an exercise regimen or come up with a healthy lifestyle that is sustainable?

People want a quick fix to enable their unhealthy lifestyle- they do not want to change it

Too many people choose various diets to lose weight. While I appreciate the effort to lose weight, many of these efforts are fads and may be inherently unhealthy. The Atkins diet is one of the common diets that many choose. It focuses less on calories, so long as carbohydrates are limited. This leads to ketosis in the body and many do lose weight while on it. Unfortunately, in some circumstances, ketosis can be unhealthy and can lead to certain organ injury. Many use this diet temporarily to lose weight, get to a lower pants or dress size and once they do, they return to their previous diet. When they gain weight again, they go back to the temporary high fat diet/low carb diet again. This back and forth or yo-yoing of weight is not healthy. People need to find a healthy diet that will help them achieve a healthy weight that is sustainable. A diet they can stick to forever that allows them to maintain a healthy weight, take in necessary nutrients and maintain a healthier existence. If you use a diet that requires you to go back and forth to maintain a weight, or depend on medications to maintain a weight, that is likely unhealthy and possibly unsafe. Many choose to undergo surgery in order to control their weight. They have given up and concede that they do not have the willpower to control their food intake or weight. While many of these people do lose significant weight after surgery, many of them later regain the weight. This adds credence to the argument that there is no easy fix that does not involve changing one's behavior and making better choices.

Non-Compliance

Many patients do not follow physician instructions. Common examples include diabetics who do not take their diabetic medicine, do not check their blood glucose, do not engage in reasonable exercise regimens or do not follow a diabetic diet and continue to eat foods high in sugars/carbohydrates. Whether these patients are in denial, are rebelling against having the disease, do not think it matters, do not believe they will get sick or simple do not care, they choose to do things that will make their conditions worse and likely lead to poor health, heart attacks, strokes, blindness, kidney failure, amputations and possible death. These same people choose to continue smoking despite repeated warnings of the additional risk of smoking in people with diabetes i.e. worsening infections, blindness, loss of limbs, heart attacks, etc.

Those with congestive heart failure often ignore diet recommendations and restrictions and continue to eat foods high in sodium and causes more fluid retention and worsening symptoms. Those with heart disease may choose not to take their blood pressure medications, continue to smoke or even neglect taking prescribed anticoagulants (blood thinners) increasing their risk for a heart attack. Patients with a stent in their coronary arteries are more likely to have a sudden heart attack or sudden death from a clot or blockage if they fail to take their blood thinners.

It is sometimes hard to explain human behavior. There are many reasons why people do what they do or do not do what they should. Reasons can include a lack of understanding, a lack of resources, stubbornness, loss of control on one's life and giving up, an indifference, a feeling of worthlessness of life, bad judgment or many others. In a sense it matters what the reason but in another sense it does not matter. The bottom line is regardless of why people do not do what they should, if they do not change their behavior and make better decisions, they and their health will continue to suffer, and they will continue to have bad outcomes. Remember the combustible engine automobile example? If one does not put gasoline in the tank and they run out of gas, it doesn't matter why they did not put gas in the car or truck, it only matters that they ran out of gas and that the engine will not run or start. One can make every excuse they want but it does not matter, the car will not run. The same could be said about the human body. One can make all kinds of excuses or give very compelling reasons why they do not do what they should. But, if they do not do what is necessary, they will likely suffer and continue to suffer. We must prevent bad things from happening and not wait until they happen. This is not being mean, cruel or insensitive, it is called being honest. We must face the truth and try to do things differently so we can improve people's health and make our health and our current healthcare system better.

Accountability: Incentives & Disincentives

Incentives, disincentives and consequences may be effective in changing people's behaviors. Some may call this tough love, others may call it accountability, while others may call it reality. Just as incentives and disincentives can help change how the healthcare complex players behave, they can also affect the decisions, behaviors and actions of patients and the public.

One would think that people would have the ultimate incentive to live healthy and make good choices: better health and avoiding pain, poor health and suffering. Unfortunately, this is not enough. As discussed, many patients make poor choices and indulge in many activities that they know are unhealthy. While we should always try to understand the reasons why and see if there is opportunity to help people make better choices through education, counseling and other resources, other incentives may be more effective. Surprisingly to anyone who truly understands the value of good health, financial incentives and disincentives can be effective, even more effective than the risk of poor health. There are others but let us first discuss the financial incentives and disincentives.

For patients, especially those with chronic diseases, why not have a reward system to reward people for taking care of themselves? Some might ask why we should pay others to take care of themselves. They should do it without anyone doing anything since it benefits them. It is true. People should need no other incentive or motivation to make good choices and live a healthy lifestyle other than the better health and less problems they will have by doing so. But the reality is, people are not perfect. Many are broken. People often make bad choices. Some may argue, if people choose to be unhealthy, then tough luck; it is their problem. Others may say, no matter what, we must forgive people, or look past their poor choices, and help no matter what. They should not be penalized. Perhaps somewhere in the middle may be the right answer. We certainly do not want to reinforce poor behavior or choices as that will most likely lead to continued poor choices and behavior or even worse behavior. This may be part of the reason why our current healthcare system is in the poor state that it is currently in. We also do not want to turn our backs and neglect patients or the problems we currently face in the current broken healthcare system. They are people. As a caring society, it is natural to forgive and want to help others.

Another point is that when people make poor choices that result in poor health or complications of their conditions, it not only affects that person but also affects society. There are significant financial costs. It costs the employer in higher healthcare costs and lower productivity, the family in stress and possible financial losses from lost productivity of the "breadwinner" and it costs society by using resources to pay for treatment and care. These costs can be much higher than what it would cost to incentivize good choices and healthier behaviors. This applies to healthy people as well. Keeping people healthy and reinforcing good choices that results in good health, benefits us all. Disincentivizing poor choices, before people have poor health and become a drain on society, is also important. It will prevent future illness, disease, expenses and suffering.

One possible model might be to look at what the average amount spent annually on every person in the last 5 or 10 years. We could also look at specific high use individuals and assign an average cost. Create a reward system that if the individual can reduce the costs of their care, he will receive a credit or check for 10-20% of the savings. Another way of doing it would be to identify specific items or behaviors that contribute to better health and reward people for complying with them i.e. stop smoking, follow diabetic diet that keep their hemoglobin A1C (HGB A1C), a blood test that measures how well blood glucose is controlled over time i.e. below a designated target, maintaining a certain weight range, maintaining a healthy exercise regimen, etc. Of course, there would have to be some way to verify compliance and other metrics that could be determined. The idea is that even though many can argue that we should not have to pay people to do what benefits them, it may be in everyone's interest to do so. It may change behavior and help people make better choices that lead to better health, lower healthcare costs, lose less time from work, lead to a higher quality of life and more productivity, then it is money well spent. Even if 25-50% of the savings are used to pay "rewards/incentives" and costs associated with the plan, still 50-75% of the savings are saved by whoever is currently paying it i.e. the patient, the employer, the taxpayer. This has the potential for savings billions upon billions of dollars each year and more importantly making people feel better, healthier and preventing unnecessary suffering.

Earlier, I stated that the average employee family insurance plan costs on average about $19,000 to $20,000 per year. Employer provided health insurance typically accounts for most of all private insurance. According to the Kaiser Family Foundation, approximately 152 million people are insured by employer-sponsored insurance plans.[93] So, if the costs are reduced by only 20% that is a potential savings of about $4,000 per family plan per employee per year. The employee could get a year-end bonus of $1,000, $1,500 or even $2,000 just for keeping themselves healthy. Of course, there are the other benefits to employees and their families' such as staying out of the hospital, saving what they would have spent on cigarettes when they decide to quit smoking, enjoying one's health and the things that can be done when one is healthy.

Another consideration is charging people for poor choices i.e. disincentives. If people choose to smoke, not follow diets, not exercise and make other choices that are known to contribute to, or worsen certain health conditions, lead to poor health or cause higher expenses to care for them, those individuals should have to pay a penalty. Before anyone objects calling this discrimination or unfair, stop and understand why we would want to this. It has nothing to do with discrimination for things that cannot be changed, it is only for bad choices and decisions. It has to do with people being allowed to make choices and when bad choices are made, there are consequences. Such is life. If we continue to find reasons why we cannot do things to get people to choose a healthy way of living, excusing the public's poor decisions and choices, then we are hurting them and hurting society. No one is making anyone do anything. No one is stopping anyone from making their own choices, good or bad. What I am saying is that there are consequences to bad choices, and we should no longer give people free passes or ignore their behavior. We should not reward bad behavior or look for excuses for them. We should not teach people how to be victims but instead encourage and empower them to make better choices and be healthy. That is what is right and best for the patient and the public.

If someone with diabetes smokes and does not follow diet requirements and their blood glucose remains at an unhealthy level, that person will have a 25% poor health penalty assessed to their health plan and it will be deducted from his paycheck. While this may seem harsh, sometimes "tough love" is necessary. Before anyone says this is not fair, his poor choices will likely cost him, his employer or society far more in future health related expenses. Why shouldn't someone have to pay more for something that costs more? Sometimes people need motivation to help themselves. If we stop coddling people who do bad things and make bad choices, we will be helping them in the long run. We will also be helping others by setting an example showing poor and unhealthy behavior will be penalized, not rewarded. Looking past people's mistakes and poor judgment may have good intentions but unfortunately it has resulted in poor results and is not helping the problem. In fact, looking past people's mistakes may be making things even worse. People must have some responsibility for themselves and accept the consequences of their actions. In this model, people will have consequences based on their actions, choices and health results. Good consequences for good choices and health; negative consequences for poor choices that result or contribute to poor health.

There are endless financial models with various goals and incentives and disincentives that can be custom designed as best seen fit by the patient, public, employer, government or insurer. There are also, non-financial factors that could be used. For example, if people do not comply with a physician's recommendation, that physician could choose to bar that patient from their practice without any consequences. If physicians did this and a patient continues to not comply with various physicians' treatment or care plans, that patient may find that at some point, they will not be able to have a physician. Before we say that is not fair to patients, we must remember that would only be the case if patients repeatedly choose to make bad decisions or not comply. Perhaps patients would stop taking for granted that the public has physicians willing to help patients, even those patients who choose not to follow the recommendations of their treating physicians. Choices have consequences. Of course, the criteria for compliance would have to be determined. For example, if the patient was non-compliant based strictly on defiance or convenience, not because of factors beyond the patient's control. But I would caution not to allow excuses to qualify as legitimate reasons not to penalize people for making poor choices and living unhealthy. Physicians are willing and able to help people who want help, are willing to be helped and will be compliant with their treatment plan. The reality is that many physicians are even willing to and do help people who do not follow the physician's recommendations or advice.

Parents of children must be held accountable for their poor choices that contribute to poor health in their children. Smoking, feeding unhealthy food to their children, and condoning or not opposing unhealthy behaviors should not be tolerated. There is no excuse for a parent not looking after, and acting in, the best interest of their children. No one is claiming parenting is easy, at least being a good and responsible parent. As a society, we should no longer look past or try to excuse poor choices of parents that adversely affect children i.e. tobacco use, condoning or not intervening if their children smoke or vape, drug use, alcohol abuse, unsafe home conditions. These parents are jeopardizing the health and safety of their children and we must hold parents accountable. No one is advocating dictating how a parent raises their children in terms of values, religion, etc. But when one smokes at home or elsewhere and wears smoke impregnated clothing home that affects a small child's breathing, or has opioids or other dangerous medications (legal or illicit) that children easily gain access to or neglect or abuse children, then these parents need to have incentives and disincentives to influence behavior. That could take the form of financial, legal or jail time penalties. If the parents will not protect helpless and dependent children, someone needs to.

The same applies to care providers. If someone is the guardian of another who is incapacitated, unable or incapable of caring for themselves and dependent upon another, then that guardian has certain responsibilities to act in best interest of that dependent person and make good choices for them. If the care provider does not, there needs to be negative consequences i.e. disincentives, that might help persuade them to make better choices in the future and lead to better health and quality of life for the dependent person the care provider is responsible to look after.

People should have free choice but must be held responsible for their decisions and choices

Government could link patient choices to other government benefits. If a person chooses to make bad health related decisions that is known to, or has high correlation to being unhealthy, then the person may be penalized by losing certain benefits. Whether loss of subsidized cell phone service or reduction or loss other subsidies, the idea is to provide the person incentives to make better choices and disincentives to discourage bad choices. Again, no one is forcing anyone to do anything. We encourage people to make their own better-informed decisions. They have the choice to make good ones and bad ones. There may be circumstances that make it hard to make the right choice, but ultimately people must be held responsible for their decisions and choices. The difference is we must hold people accountable for the choices they make and see to it that the consequences associated with bad choices and unhealthy lifestyles occur. Of course, there should be good consequences too, a.k.a. rewards, for people to choose better, live healthier and ultimately be better off than they are under the current healthcare system.

The public needs to hold their elected governmental officials accountable. The public needs to communicate with their senators, congressmen and local representatives and tell them the issues that they are having with healthcare. These officials are the people who make the laws. These same people are the ones who are supposed to serve the people, not rule them. These legislators and government officials work for the public, are paid by taxpayers' dollars and need to be reminded of this, if necessary. Write letters, send e-mails, call their offices. Tell them what is happening in the real world and how it is affecting us, the people they are supposed to represent. Tell them what we want them to do and what we expect and want to happen. One might be surprised; many will be receptive and even appreciative. Many want to do the right thing; this helps them be better-informed and accomplish doing "good." Even if one is skeptical or even cynical of whether their voice matters, look at it another way. Even if the representatives in government don't care about us and only care about themselves, if they believe that a topic such as healthcare is important enough to the public, that it will affect how people vote, it suddenly matters to them. Even if, and maybe especially if, they are selfish and only concerned with getting re-elected, they realize if enough people want change or a certain thing to happen and are willing to vote in the next election to remove them if they do not satisfy the voters, the senator or representative will now understand that it is in their best interest to do what the people want. They will "obey" the will of the people or risk being kicked out of office in the next election i.e. suffer the consequences of not doing what the people want. This is how the system works or is supposed to work. We should not take for granted the power that we have as citizens of this great country. We have the right, and some say the duty, to let our representatives hear our opinion and help make our healthcare system great.

Chapter 11 Talking Points:

- People are the most important and most influential part of a great healthcare system.
- Simple things like hand washing, avoiding those who may be ill, covering our mouths when we cough or sneeze, etc. can potentially prevent illness and more suffering than can expensive antibiotics
- Things we take for granted like garbage pick-up, clean drinking water, indoor plumbing, sanitation etc. prevent more illness and save more lives than doctors and medications.
- If someone could convince everyone to never smoke again, he or she might be responsible for saving more lives and preventing more suffering than anyone in the history of the work.
- The diet and lifestyle of a person may have a bigger impact on their health than genetics
- Diet is human fuel. If we eat healthy, we are more likely to be healthy.
- People have unrealistic expectations. They want a pill to fix whatever ailment or problem they have instead of eating healthier, making smarter decisions and living healthier lifestyles.
- People have a responsibility to learn more about healthcare and how to improve their own health
- No one should be forced to do anything. People should have the right to make their own choices.
- There need to be incentives to encourage good choices and disincentives to discourage bad choices.
- People must be accountable for their choices and actions.
- There are consequences to everyone's decisions, choices and actions.
- Instead of worrying about being politically correct to the detriment of our health, we need to be honest with ourselves and one another.
- Honesty demonstrates respect to another individual.

Edward Shaheen, M.D.

Chapter Twelve:
DIET, MEDICAL MARTS & SIMPLE PACKAGE LABELING

We have already introduced creative ideas and innovative concepts such as Direct Care Organizations, Price-Quality Disclosures, Policy Weakness Disclosures, Lifetime Health Policies, Hybrid Health-Life Insurance Policies, Medical Menus and Medication Menus. Later in this chapter, I will introduce Healthy Marts and D-Meals. But first, let's talk about the "fuel" we put into our bodies, our diet.

What is healthy and unhealthy depends on who you ask. Many will say that a diet that is low in fat and cholesterol is healthy. Others will say diets that do not contain high amounts of sugars; others will say avoiding fried foods. Others would say one that minimizes or eliminates processed foods. Others will say a diet high in fiber. Others say eating diets with lots of fruits and vegetables. Others will say eating natural foods. Others will say eating organic. Others will say fresh foods. The point is that there is a lot a variation of what people, even experts, believe is healthy or unhealthy. Some argue health is determined by genetics and diet doesn't matter. While genetics can and do play a role, most agree that genetics is not the only factor that matters. Diet plays an important role in our overall health. Some believe diet is more important than genetics. Many people believe that a diet high in red meats is not good. Some state red meat of any kind is not ideal and suggest substituting other meats instead. Still others believe meat of any kind may be harmful. The push, by some, of plant-based proteins is becoming more accepted and popular and is something that should be investigated further.

About 80,000,000,000 animals die, or are killed, each year for food just in the United States

Some are moving more towards plant-based proteins for humane beliefs. As people become aware of animal suffering, the cruel, "inhumane" and terrible conditions in which many animals are raised, treated and slaughtered in the food industry, they attempt to avoid eating meat as a means of decreasing demand for meat and the suffering it causes. By doing so, the hope is to end, or at least, decrease the cruel and horrible conditions billions of animals must live in until they are killed for human and other animal consumption. In 2008, 8,560,000,000 land animals and 71 billion sea animals were killed, or died, for food in the United States alone.[94] According to Animal Matters website, during an average, non-vegan, person's lifetime that lives in a developed country, each person will consume about 7,000 animals. Over 70 billion animals are reared worldwide for food each year. Approximately 2/3 of all farm animals reared worldwide are done so on a factory farm; 99% of farm animals reared in the US are reared on a factory farm. Every day, over 160 million farm animals around the world are transported to a slaughterhouse.[95] Books, documentaries, websites, organizations, etc. discuss the cruel and sad ways animals are raised, housed, fed, slaughtered and treated. We will not go into the details in this book of all the animal suffering but if you need further convincing, they you may want to do your own research or an internet search on the subject and reach your own conclusion.

Some are choosing to avoid meat due to the unsanitary conditions in which our meat is raised, slaughtered, processed or packaged. There have been many recalls of beef and chicken products because of health and safety concerns. One of the reasons has been due to E Coli contamination, which is the name of one of the bacteria found in feces. The DailyMail.com reported "Consumer Reports tested 300 packages of ground beef from 103 stores in 26 cities across the country in order to test the prevalence of bacteria in the meat" and every sample tested showed fecal contamination.[96] For clarity, fecal contamination is another way of saying that there is stool within the ground beef that people are buying to eat and feed to their families. Stool bacteria was in in every sample.

All ground beef samples had fecal contamination

Others are moving towards plant-based proteins for environment reasons. Animal agriculture and meat consumption contribute considerably to global warming. It is reported that animal agriculture accounts for 14%-18% of all greenhouse gas emissions.[97] It takes 10 times as much energy from fossil fuels to produce 1 calorie from animal sources as it does to produce one calorie from plant foods. Since the 1970's, 20% of the Amazon Rain Forrest has been destroyed and 80% of the destroyed portion is being used for livestock. That is an area the size of the state of California. The world's cattle eat enough grain to feed 8.7 billion people. The amount of grain used just to feed cattle could feed every single human on the planet and have enough extra to feed another 2 billion.[98] If humans adopted plant-based diets, there would be plenty of food. Enough food to eliminate world hunger. Humans would have a much smaller carbon footprint and cause much less damage to the environment by going vegan.

The world's cattle eat enough grain to feed 8.7 billion people

Depending on your beliefs, the move towards a vegan diet because of animal rights and treatment reasons and because of environment reasons may be viewed as admirable, honorable and responsible. Regardless of one's belief, from a health perspective, it is hard to make a strong scientific argument that moving towards vegan and away from diets consisting of lots of meats and animal proteins is harmful or a bad thing. Of course, there can be a discussion regarding the jobs or financial consequences of eliminating or shrinking the meat industry i.e. farms, slaughtering houses, processing plants, packaging, etc., or the concern that people would not have a means of getting enough proteins or B vitamins. Without going into a long discussion of these points, we will keep it limited to saying that the financial impact could be offset with other industries and conscious benefits of no longer treating living creatures in cruel and inhumane ways. Similar arguments were made with the introduction of modern equipment into the farming industry, it will significantly reduce the required amount of human labor eliminating jobs and causing financial consequences. Farming still went forward with the modern equipment and society is better off because of it. Many would even call this progress. Money is important to many for many reasons, but we always must decide at what costs and look at many factors, not just money. There is also a potential huge financial benefit of shifting away from meat we will soon discuss. As for the protein and B12 argument, there are other ways to obtain enough protein without the need for meat. To illustrate, there are vegan body builders who are quite "bulked up." Another interesting fact is that some of the largest land animals such as the elephant, rhino and gorilla eat diets consisting primarily or exclusively of plants.[99] Unlike what some may believe, meat is not necessary for humans to get enough proteins in their diet.

Some argue that there is no environment issue. There are those on both sides of the issue of climate change and protecting the environment. If you are a believer in climate change and protecting the environment, it is a no brainer to avoid animal protein for environment purposes. According to the director of *What the Health*, animal agriculture or "raising animals for food produces more greenhouse gases than the entire transportation sector."[100] With few, or any, exceptions, going vegan helps the environment. It is hard to make a strong, substantiated argument that going vegan will hurt the environment. It one does not buy the environment argument or does not care about it; the environment argument will not sway you anyway.

From an evolutionary and "design" standpoint, humans are not meant to be carnivores

For a moment, let's pretend that there are no animal or environment reasons to stop eating meat for the sake of discussion. There is at least one other, very important reason to cut out meat and go towards a vegan diet: your health. More and more people are beginning to understand the health benefits of protein-based protein diets. While, we could literally write a book about plant-based protein diets, we will simply say that it is believed that by eliminating all animal products from our diets, we could potentially improve our population health by an unbelievable amount. How much? Some argue that we could reduce healthcare costs by as much as 70-80% if everyone adopted a plant-based diet.[101] This is because there is some data and/or belief to suggest that animal protein i.e. meat, could be responsible for many illnesses and diseases including but not limited to cancer, cardiovascular disease including heart attacks and strokes, diabetes, auto-immune diseases, Alzheimer's, etc. It is thought that eating meat causes inflammation in our bodies and such inflammation at the microscopic level may contribute to or cause many human illnesses and diseases.[102] If this is even close to accurate, this is earthshattering news. By changing our diets and eating a more healthy diet, as defined by avoiding animal-based proteins, humans could become much healthier, avoid hundreds of billions of dollars of healthcare costs each year and save as much as 70% or more of the $3-4 trillion a year we spend in healthcare and most importantly prevent so much human suffering. If we could save 70% a year on healthcare, we could potentially save TRILLIONS a year in the United States alone. This should dwarf or offset any loss from the current lucrative and profitable meat industry.

From an evolutionary and common-sense standpoint, humans really were not meant to be carnivores, or meat eaters. At least, one can make the argument that humans were not meant to not consume meat on a frequent basis or consume a large percentage of our calories as meat. Compare the shape of the human face, the location of the nose and mouth and the shape and size of man's teeth. Our canine teeth are nothing like the canine teeth of carnivores such as a dogs, coyotes or wolves. Carnivore animal mouths are pointed. Their mouths, teeth and faces are ideal for biting, ripping and tearing a chuck of meat and flesh of another animal. The human face, mouth and teeth are not. We have relatively flat faces and our teeth are not "designed" to rip and tear flesh and meat. The human canine teeth are very similar in size and function as our lateral incisors and premolars. There may be dentists who say this is an exaggeration but the difference between a human canine tooth and an animal carnivore's is impressive. Animals' heads, mouths and teeth are lower to the ground as they do not stand and walk in the upright position as the Homo sapiens species does. Humans have arms that can reach and incredible tools at the ends of them called fingers and the opposing thumbs. The amazing opposable thumb that separate us and enable us to do amazing things that fellow animals cannot do. Our "design" is for "picking" things up and placing them into our mouths i.e. fruits, berries, and vegetables. Few animals do this and the ones that do, typically pick up vegetation, not meat, and place it in their mouths.

One may bring up that "early" man ate meat, and this is true. It is very likely that this was a relatively infrequent event. Perhaps once a month or even once a week, should they be so lucky to catch an animal or stumble upon a non-devoured animal. Yet, I am not aware that anyone believes that man ate meat each day, every day and several times a day as humans currently do. Let's face it, prehistoric man did not have McDonald's, Burger King, Wendy's, Chick-fil-A, BBQ joints, KFC, etc. or the convenience of ranchers, factory farms, butcher shops, supermarkets, etc.

80% of all antibiotics produced in the United States are used for animal agriculture[103]

Add to that, the meat we currently eat is often processed and consists of animals who were fed antibiotics, steroids or other un-natural chemicals. Surprisingly, 80% of all antibiotics produced in the United States are used for animal agriculture.[104] Antibiotics, along with hormones and other chemicals are used on the animals that people eat yet we are not 100% sure of all the harmful effects that they have on young children and adults.

As I touched on earlier. Defining a healthy diet is difficult. Perhaps a vegan diet is what may turn out to be what a healthy diet is. Doctors, dieticians, special societies, etc. argue or cannot agree on what is healthy or unhealthy. Even if they did, would what they agree on be accurate? There is so much information and conflicting information out there. It is unclear if that is just the way it is or intentional to create doubt and keep the public confused. This might sound like a conspiracy theory. The meat industry and anyone who benefits from the way things are would not want things to change. There is a lot of money at stake. It is estimated that the worldwide beef industry alone is about a trillion dollar per year business.[105]

The World Health Organization (WHO) rates bacon as a carcinogen in the same category that it rates cigarettes, asbestos and plutonium.[106] But is this common knowledge? The WHO "declared that processed meat is definitely a carcinogen, with the most powerful link to colon cancer."[107] Red meat is particularly of concern. "The strongest, but still limited, evidence for an association with eating red meat is for colorectal cancer."[108] It has been stated that certain European studies demonstrate that meat may be a cause, or increase the chances of developing, diabetes mellitus but does the ADA mention this in their literature or on their website?[109] The WHO has stated that there is evidence that there is an association between red meat and colorectal cancer, pancreatic cancer and prostate cancer. There is also evidence of links with pancreatic cancer and prostate cancer. It is estimated that for every 50 grams, less than 2 ounces, of processed meat consumed daily, there is an increased risk of colorectal cancer by 18%.[110] The beef industry, processing plants, slaughterhouses or supermarkets do a poor job communicating this information to the general public.

In the 2011 Netflix Documentary *Forks over Knives*, Dr. Caldwell Esselstyn, MD, of the Cleveland Clinic provides fascinating statistics regarding cardiovascular disease in Norway before, during and after

Nazi Germany took over most of Europe during WWII.[111] Prior to 1939, the rate of cardiovascular disease in Norway was high and consistent with many other developed countries that had "western diets" that consisted of significant amounts of meat. At the end of 1939 and beginning of 1940, when Germany exerted its military dominance, there was a significant decline in meat consumption in Norway, likely because the Nazis diverted the prized meat and dairy to Germany and Germans. At about the same time, the rate of cardiovascular disease in Norway dropped suddenly. It remained low during WWII but once the Germans were defeated in 1945, when meat and dairy once again became common in the Norwegian diet, the rate of cardiovascular disease shot back up to pre-war levels. This is consistent with meat and/or dairy being strong risk factors for cardiovascular disease. As a physician and someone who can be critical of scientific studies, such a "study" seems rather convincing to me. Why? Unlike studies where people may choose to eliminate meat and dairy in order to try to be healthy, where one could argue that if there is an improvement in health, it could be because of reducing meat and dairy or it could be from other factors. Such factors as consuming less calories, exercising, cutting out smoking, etc. One could argue that someone who wants to be healthy does other things that are healthy, and those other things could be the cause of better health, not just eliminating meat and dairy. But the Norwegians did not have any choice. The Germans took the meat and cows, so there was little to no meat or dairy for the Norwegians to consume. All Norwegians, not just those who wanted to be healthy but everyone, even the Norwegians with unhealthy lifestyles were affected. Thus, what happened in Norway eliminates some of the biases that might occur in some scientific studies. As a physician who has been taught to be critical of studies and evidence, this example was powerful to me.

Ask representatives of the meat and dairy companies or others who stand to lose hundreds of billions of dollars in revenue if people cut back on or eliminated meat and dairy, and they are likely to deny that meat or dairy is unhealthy. Perhaps some may concede that one should limit the amount that a person eats i.e. moderation or use common sense but not defining what that means. They may also try to cast doubt on any research or concerns voiced by health experts. This casting of doubt is often all that humans need to continue doing what they know deep down, or at least should know, is bad for them. This brings up memories of the tobacco industry many years ago. What did the tobacco company do for decades? They denied that cigarette smoking caused cancer, heart disease, lung disease and many diseases. This was even though the tobacco companies had knowledge and their own research showed that cigarette smoking in fact does cause many terrible illnesses and diseases. For decades, tobacco companies' representatives casted doubt about the dangers of tobacco use. When they were required to place warnings, the "warnings" stated that cigarette smoking may be harmful. It was many years after cigarettes were first sold to the public that they finally provided the required "surgeon general" warning. By that time, it is unclear if it made any difference to current smokers or children who had not yet begin to smoke. In the 2017 Netflix Documentary *What the Health*, Dr. Michael Greger, MD, discusses the "famous tobacco memo" that was reported as stating "doubt is our product."[112] If the tobacco companies could introduce doubt, they could confuse the public and that was all that was needed to allow cigarette sales to thrive.

Without accusing anyone of anything, I am just asking you to think. Do your own research and investigating. Ask questions. Do not assume what someone says is true just because they say so. Others may be biased and trying to protect what is important to them i.e. livelihood, financial support or profits. Everyone should protect what is important to them including their health and the health of their family and loved ones. Given that our health may be at stake, it is not worth spending some time looking into it, finding unbiased information and learning more?

Determining what is healthy for the average person can be confusing. From a population health standpoint, an employer who pays for their employees' healthcare standpoint, an insurer trying to minimize utilization standpoint or even a person trying to stay healthy to avoid pain and suffering standpoint, it would benefit all of us to stay healthy. If eating healthy helps us get or stay healthy, it would behoove us individually and as a society to eat healthy. While some might argue that the data is not conclusive, most everyone would admit that diet does indeed matter and that we could improve our health from eating a healthy diet. On the same note, most would agree that it is worth trying to learn what diet is healthy. Perhaps doing studies with people eating what a consensus may believe is healthy. Perhaps different groups trying various variations of what is thought to be healthy and then looking objectively at the data. Objectively meaning trying to eliminate bias. Of course, eliminate as much research and study population bias and the bias of those who stand to benefit from certain results i.e. having researchers independent of the meat or dairy industry that receive no financial support from them or their lobbyists, etc. We want to find the truth of what will help us be healthy, no matter what the findings or who will win or lose from it. Then people can make their own, better informed choices, based on accurate, unbiased data.

The concept of Healthy Marts (HM) could be developed and implemented. It is just one idea to make things simpler and to improve our diet and health. We really do not have to wait for research to begin to make smarter and better decisions. We should still do research and analyze the data that exists and that will be produced with time, but we do not have to wait years for the results before we try to make better decisions. If it makes sense and you believe you can make better choices, why wait? Many smokers probably believed and knew deep down that smoking tobacco was harmful even before Big Tobacco admitted it. Yet these smokers did not act on this knowledge or feeling. They continued to smoke and caused more harm to their health and the health of those around them. Healthy marts could eliminate much of the confusion associated with trying to figure out what foods are healthy or what foods may contain and whether it is appropriate for an illness or disease. Healthy marts would make finding a diagnosis-based diet, easier to find. These meals are called Diagnosis Diets (DD) or

Diagnosis Meals (D-Meals).

Clarence "Kelly" Johnson is credited with the design principal of "Keep It Simple Stupid" (K.I.S.S.). He was an engineer at Lockheed Skunk Works that worked with the US Navy in the early 1960's that helped to design very complex things including the Blackbird spy plane.[113] The idea was that no matter how complex the design may be, the plane or other item i.e. engine, needed to be simple enough that the average Navy mechanic could work on it. By keeping it simple, more people will likely understand and be able to make use of and contribute to the project or efforts. The same concept that Kelly Johnson had with keeping things simple even when it came to complex naval spy aircraft can be applied to healthcare and eating the proper diet. By keeping things simple, more people will be able to understand, or understand enough, and participate in the healthy mart program. They do not have to understand everything about it but will understand enough to be successful at eating a diet that is "right" for them. Much of the problem with eating a healthy diet is that eating healthy can be complicated and confusing. With all the marketing, labeling and packaging in today's food industry, the consumer may believe that they are eating healthy because the product says "healthy," "natural," "low-calorie" or "recommended." But the product may not be what the consumer believes it to be and could be unhealthy. People could benefit now from making better choices, even if it ultimately turns out not to be the absolute best decision. If we later determine that other diet combinations are optimal, these new options could be incorporated into the healthy marts that are already established. We can use the best information we have available at this time and start the process.

So, what is a "Healthy Mart" and what would one look like? A healthy mart is a shopping location, standalone or within another facility, where food items are labeled in a simple, easy to understand manner. In addition to the typical list of ingredients on the package that is currently used, D-Meals would have color coded packaging and have a numbering system to help make selecting healthy and appropriate food for people to eat a meal specific to their diagnosis easier. In addition, a certain design could be used to further distinguish the D-Meals. For example, green, and numbers ranging from 1000-1999, labeled items are healthy in general i.e. no processed foods and a balance of protein, carbohydrates and fat. Red, and numbers 2000-2999, items are healthy and may be of interest in heart patients, congestive heart patients or anyone with cardiovascular disease concerns. Yellow, or 3000-3999, items are healthy and of interest to those treated, diagnosed or at risk for diabetes. Dialysis or renal patients could have another color and number range. Cancer another. Those trying to lose weight another. The color-coded system is one method, numbering is another code system, a combination of the two is probably the best. Having numbering as a component would certainly help individuals who may be color blind. Including color coding could prove helpful to those who cannot read or who have sub-optimal vision and unable to see small print or numbers. It is easiest to recognize a color, even more than a design or what something says.

D-meals can make complying with diet restrictions easier to do

Complete meals could be packaged according to a person's medical diagnosis or whatever other factor that would be useful. If it has its own color and number, it can easily be distinguished from other meals that may not be appropriate. These D-meals could simplify food shopping for patients with various medical diagnoses or anyone who has special dietary requirements. Given technology, and the preference and convenience of the public, healthy marts would also have an online presence. People could shop by categories i.e. medical diagnoses or diet goals, make purchases and have their diagnosis specific groceries delivered to their homes as a one-time delivery or on a subscription, regularly occurring, schedule. So, if someone is a diabetic, they could go to the Healthy Mart or online and easily find single serving meals made especially for diabetics by looking for the yellow colored packaging or the number between 3000-3999. The point is that it will be simpler and thus much easier for patients to be compliant with their dietary requirements.

For example, when someone is first diagnosed with diabetes or when a diabetic is discharged from the hospital and instructed to follow a diabetic diet, does that person really know what that means? Can they have cereal? Can they have a sandwich or eat bread and if so, how much and what kind? Can a congestive heart failure patient eat soup? What about pasta? Does the food have to be fresh or can it be pre-made or frozen? The point is that it is complicated to know even for a well-educated and sophisticated individual. Many patients are not well educated or sophisticated. Many people cannot see well enough to read the label contents. Many people don't have the time to do the research. Keep it simple!

By having a simple labeling system, color and number coded, the diabetic would know that by choosing a yellow colored and numbered package/stripe/D-Meal logo, they would know that it meets recommended dietary requirements and restrictions for a diabetic in terms of calories, carbohydrates, nutrition, etc. I.e. baked chicken and vegetables 3025 in a yellow colored D-Meal Logo package. This way a diabetic could choose from various meals and know that it was a reasonable option for diabetics because it was yellow and had a number on it between 3000 and 3999. The diabetic would not have to struggle with trying to research each product off the shelf by reading ingredients and determining if it is allowed or not, doing the math or other potentially complicating factors that might currently lead to diabetics just giving up and eating whatever meal that is available or least expensive. By using this system, if it truly increases compliance, patients would be more likely to remain healthy and avoid complications of their disease and costly ER visits, hospital admissions or re-admissions. The same would apply to patients with other medical conditions i.e. congestive heart failure, heart disease, hypertension, kidney disease, etc.

Of course, the packaging in this new simplified labeling system would still have disclosures of ingredients, calories, amount of protein and sugars, nutritional value, etc. as required and for anyone who wanted to know. We would recommend avoiding using subjective and potentially misleading marketing terms such as "healthy", "low-calorie" or such but to try to maintain consistency and objectivity.

Healthy marts could be their own standalone stores or supermarkets or could be contained within existing supermarkets. The stand-alone model has the advantage of being recognized as places that only have healthy food. To avoid any confusion, before being able to market themselves as a healthy mart, the healthy mart would have to meet certain requirements to help protect the public from confusion. For example, items that are not "healthy" or that could be misleading would not be allowed to be sold in Healthy Mart stores. The idea is to help make it easier for a person to make better choices. If located in the healthy mart space, the public could be more confident that any food purchased in a Healthy Mart meets certain criteria and is consistent with the type of diet recommended by their doctor or nutritionist as indicated by its color or numeric coding.

One drawback to the healthy mart concept is that it would be much more expensive to start an entirely new business, with its own building, staff and all the expenses involved to only sell healthy food. Sounds ironic as this implies that one needs to sell unhealthy food to be financially successful. Unfortunately, there is a lot of money and profit in foods that are unhealthy or are not the healthiest. Look at all the profits and revenues from "sugar-water" sales of icon brands such as Coke, Pepsi, Gatorade and other national and international brands that sell fat loaded, sugar loaded and processed foods. Even beverages thought to be "good" for you such as orange juice and other fruit drinks contain lots of, or are artificially flavored with, sugars and/or other items that are not the healthiest to have in the amounts contained in the products. Added to this is many people do not just drink one but often drink more than one soda or other high sugar drink. Some argue that diet drinks avoid this problem. While it is true that they avoid the sugar or calorie problem, diet drinks have their own health risks and concerns and are not considered to be healthy. Some believe they are unhealthier than the sugar containing drinks they often replace.

This new labeling system of D-Meals would hopefully prevent the confusion that exists today. For example, there may be a product that is marketed as "low calorie" and is labeled as such on the package or in marketing efforts. Yet, the product may contain calories much in excess of the recommendations for good health. The low-calorie statement may refer to one serving which might only be 2 ounces but there are 12 ounces in the container. A consumer might assume that the low calorie applies to the entire container and not realize that there are 6 servings in the container. Whether or not the manufacturer or advertising intends to deceive or mislead the consumer really is not the point. That is an entirely different discussion. The point here is that the consumer makes unhealthy choices when they believe they are making healthy choices. The result: the person's health suffers, and this is bad. Another simple concept within the healthy mart and healthy packaging concept would be to package single servings per package. Again, this would simplify things. One package, one serving. One could make the argument that people should read the label and know better. History has shown us that this is often not the case. In an ideal world people would but the reality is that people are not perfect and instead of blaming them, even though people do have to accept responsibility, we can do things to make things easier for people to make better choices and eat healthier, more appropriate diets. Unless people know better or have other, more compelling reasons to change, it is hard for people to make better choices.

Another option would be to have a healthy mart department within an existing supermarket. It could be separate from the rest of the store with its own "entrance" that distinguishes it as its own area. This symbolic separation is important to give the consumer a sense of simplicity to know that anything that is purchased from this section is "healthy." Perhaps a separate entrance to this part of the supermarket from the outside or a symbolic and very conspicuous entrance, with signage, from the main supermarket making it obvious that you are entering a healthy mart. Anything here would be coded using the same simple color coded, single serving and numbered packaging. These healthy marts within a supermarket offer the advantage of being a less costly way of opening such stores compared to a separate building with its own separate staff, inventory system, etc. The drawback of healthy marts within a traditional store is there could be some confusion by the consumer or the temptation of the storeowner to put high profit, less healthy items in that area of the store that consumers might purchase. The mixing in of unhealthy, or non-D-Meals, in Healthy Marts or in Healthy Mart sections of supermarkets, should be prohibited and supermarkets owners penalized if they do not follow this rule. Regulations should be such that we prevent confusion and allow people to make informed decisions without being deceived, misled or confused, particularly with something that could affect something as important as a person's health.

Some say, if one shops only in the perimeter of a supermarket, they are more likely to buy healthier foods than if they purchase items from the middle of the store. In many cases, there is some truth to this. Many of the items in the middle contain foods that are processed, high in sugars, high in sodium, etc. The outer perimeter has the fresh fruits, vegetables and produce. But there are also items that are not necessarily the most-healthy in the perimeter either such as yogurts that can contain lots of sugars, fruit drinks with lots of sugars and artificial colors and sweeteners, meats with high fat or cholesterol and the questionable health complications of animal based proteins, etc. So, you must be careful, this "rule" of things on the perimeter of the supermarket being healthy may not be as simple as it sounds.

Assuming we agree that eating healthy is important, how do we incentivize people to do it. One hopes people would do it because it could keep them healthy. As I have discussed, human nature is not to always do the right thing. People are people. They want what they want and what the marketers have so effectively marketed to them. Education is the first step. Making things easier to understand and having protections in place to deter and penalize misleading ads, marketing and packaging is a step in the right direction. Simple labeling systems as we have already discussed. Another way to incentive better choices in diet is providing financial or other incentives to make healthier diet choices.

It might be in the interest of those who pay for healthcare or the patient's unhealthy lifestyle and choices to pay for or subsidize groceries for people so long as they are healthy. One example might be for an employer or insurer to negotiate a discount with supermarkets for anything purchased only in the healthy mart area of the store. Another would be a "credit card" or pre-paid "Healthy Card" that can only be used to purchase items in the healthy mart.

Other perks might be for employers, insurers or even hospitals to provide free delivery of these healthy mart food items to the person's home. This may be a convenience to some but could be a "game changer" for others. Some people do not have transportation and rely on others. If the others do not shop healthy, then those who rely on the transportation of these people have little to no choice as to what they buy. If their ride only shops at typical supermarkets that do not have Healthy Marts, then these people may continue to eat unhealthy even though they might want to eat better. Today the concept of food delivery is a reality. Companies such as UberEATS, Grub Hub, DoorDash, and other food delivery services, already are delivering food. Amazon and Walmart are already delivering groceries to some degree. Why not deliver healthy groceries and D-Meals too?

Another important perk might be providing a home visit. Of course, we must be cautious not to overstep our right or invade an individual's privacy, but home visits can be quite valuable. One, the patient's general health can be evaluated. Two, the person's home environment can be evaluated and could reveal factors that affect the person's health that might otherwise be unknown. For example, if a child with asthma has repeated admissions for exacerbations of his or her illness, it might be discovered that someone is smoking in the home when the home visitor sees cigarette butts or the home smells of cigarette smoke. If asked during a doctor's visit, a patient or family member of a child may deny that anyone smokes in the home. With the knowledge learned from a home visit, the cause of the child's asthma exacerbation can be addressed. Other dangers may be discovered as uncovered electrical outlets, opioid or other potentially dangerous medications not secured or locked that could be accidentally ingested by a child, or a poor living environment i.e. no heat or AC, no food in refrigerator or pantry, uncleanliness, etc.

Such "perks" to patients should be part of any hospital discharge instructions. There should be a person designated with the role to follow up with a home visit to make sure the discharged patient is doing well, was able to get the medications prescribed, is taking the medications as prescribed, is eating the proper diet, and was able to shop and buy the appropriate groceries specific to them. In fact, medications could be delivered to the patient's home if there is any question or concern as to whether the patient has transportation to the pharmacy. Home delivery should be the default method for prescriptions to be obtained unless patients choose otherwise. It is one less thing that patients will have to worry about in order to comply with their treatment and instructions. The more convenient and simple things are, the more likely the patient will be able to comply and the more likely the patient will get and stay healthy. Keep it simple. While these perks might sound excessive or expensive to some, the costs of being unhealthy can be massive. The saving from one hospitalization that can be avoided could pay for an entire year of food, home delivery or home visits. This does not consider the savings of other costs to the patient's family, lost productivity and pain and suffering that might otherwise occur. With the various new businesses such as Amazon, Uber, Lyft, etc. created by entrepreneurs and with the technological advancements such as drones becoming common, it is very possible and likely that more and more innovative and effective ways of helping people will continue to arise. Hopefully, it will be easier and less costly for the public to make better and healthier choices that will lead to better health.

Professional athletes have sports agents. Why not have Health Agents?

Health Consultants (HC), Medical Managers (MM), Health Agent and Health Advisor (HA) are essentially the same and will be used interchangeably. People have personal trainers for helping them work out. Others have motivational or life coaches to help make them more successful. Professional athletes have sports agents. Why not have Health Agents (HAs)? This person would act as a consultant, manager or agent who understands, schedules and handles just about everything related to health in order to help a person maximize health. Among other things, the HA would help people choose better suited health plans, research the quality scores of doctors and hospitals that may be needed, negotiate better rates for services, procedures and surgeries and locate better prices for needed medications. Unlike a personal trainer who might help someone work out and try to get physically fit with big muscles or a toned abdomen, the HA would manage most all aspects of the person's health. This service could be paid for by the individual, a health insurer or whomever foots the bill for healthcare expenses. The idea is that if someone can schedule and manage healthcare well, the patient will be healthier, and the HM's fee/salary will be more than covered by the savings in healthcare resulting from of staying healthy because of the HM. One might ask isn't that what a primary care physician (PCP) is supposed to do? In a sense yes. Many PCPs do in fact try their best to coordinate all aspects of health but quite honestly, it is a full-time job just to coordinate all the various aspects, let alone try to practice medicine. Plus, it is not common for PCPs to act as the patient's agent to negotiate rates and services on their behalf and help patients choose insurance plans. The PCP may find themselves in an awkward position trying to negotiate a lower rate with a hospital on behalf of a patient that the doctor may practice within, or work for. A PCP would have a conflict of interest trying to maintain objectivity negotiating better rates or terms on behalf of the patient with the patient's PCP (himself). Add to this, higher expenses that physicians incur with their practice related expenses and the way reimbursement is today, and you see physicians simple cannot do it all. In our current healthcare system, there is not enough time in the day. Physicians are asked to do so many things by government regulations or insurance companies that they end up spending less and less time with patients and more time on things that often do not directly affect one's health.

HCs can fulfill many of the roles and perform many of the tasks that physicians do, or do not have the time to do. MMs can do a lot more too. So long as someone understands the needs and is good at organizing, communications and scheduling, negotiating and has good judgment and common sense, one without a medical degree can perform this valuable role. In a sense, the MM is the "office manager" of a patient's health "office." The MM would serve many functions including but not limited to:

- Understanding the patient's health and needs, regular appointment needs, coordinating appointments with PCP, specialists and other health providers
- Knowing the patient's economic status as to what they might and might not be able to afford
- Being aware and familiar with the patient's home and/or living environment and possible challenges such as if the patient is homeless, if the person has heat, air conditioning, power and water
- Knowing if the patient has food to eat; making sure dietary needs are met including being able to afford, obtain and consume the proper meals specific for the patient's requirements

- Knowing if the patient has transportation to and from appointments, other health related providers, the grocery store and pharmacy or arranging to have groceries and/or medications delivered
- Understanding the patient's insurance plan and the particulars of that insurance to help explain to the patient
- Helping to advise or negotiate with insurers, physicians, hospitals, imaging centers, pharmacies, medical device makers, etc.
- Doing most any other function that might help a patient that a he or she may require or that may help make them healthier.

The HC's primary role is to the patient, no one else. These HCs would play an important and valuable role. HCs would be responsible for a fixed number of patients and would provide complete services. Such coaches could save thousands of dollars or more per patient per year and could potentially save hundreds of thousands of dollars to the payers of those the HC manages. HC should be paid well and incentivized based on performance i.e. good outcomes, health of the people he or she manages and savings.

It would make sense for whoever the payer is to enlist the services of a HC. For most current private insurance, that would likely be the employer. For Medicare, Medicaid and Tricare or VA related care, that would be the government. Insurers may choose to use HCs or even private citizens could choose to hire HCs. It is important that not just anyone is chosen to serve the role and that the HC is not overloaded or expected to do more than she can reasonably be expected to do effectively and efficiently. It is also important that the HC does not have conflicts of interest i.e. kickbacks, a financial interest in any entity that benefits from patients the HC "manages" related to healthcare, etc. The HC's compensation should only be from what is received serving the patient's best interest i.e. patient-obsessed©. It takes a special person with special skills to be able to do a great job. If you overload HCs, then they too will be unable to spend the necessary time to do what it takes to reach their potential in order to keep people healthy and help lower expenses.

The HC would have access to anyone or entity i.e. physician, dietician, social worker, nursing, source of medical supplies, pharmacy, transportation company, and any other resource that the person may need. The new healthcare system would have a system by which everyone at any given time could know exactly what is going on, what the status of any patient is, what is needed, what is being done to get it done and by who and in what time frame. There would also be a way of holding everyone accountable. Accountable to reward for good health/outcomes and to penalize for poor health of the person/patient. In such an arrangement, technology would play a big role and help patients have access to most any provider remotely, to track the many players in one's health and help keep everyone accountable.

Chapter 12 Talking Points:

- A person's diet may be more important to one's health than genetics
- There is evidence that red meat can contribute to the development of cancer
- Two ounces of processed meat a day increases the risk of colorectal cancer by 18%
- Bacon is a carcinogen and is rated in the same category as cigarettes, asbestos and plutonium by the World Health Organization (WHO)
- Animal agriculture accounts for 14-18% of all greenhouse gas emissions
- The world's cattle eat enough grain that could feed 8.7 billion people (more than the world's population
- In 2008, 8.5 Billion land animals and 71 Billion sea animals were killed for food in the United States alone.
- Escherichia coli a.k.a. E. coli, one of the coliform bacteria found in feces, is commonly found in meat that is sold in supermarkets intended for human consumption.

Edward Shaheen, M.D.

Chapter Thirteen:
TECHNOLOGY

Electronic Medical Records EMRs- Hospitals Inefficiencies

Electronic medical records (EMR) a.k.a. electronic health records (EHRs), touted as something that will help physicians see patients faster, may actually do the exact opposite. While advantages of EMRs include legibility and the ability to require certain information to be collected, they often miss the ability to accurately, efficiently and effectively capture a patient's history and physical exam that a physician performs and is so important in a patient's care. Often, EMRs require significantly more physician time than simple hand- writing. Prior to EMRs, an EP might have seen 30, 40 or 50 or more patients in a 12-hour shift and been able to accurately document the patient's chief complaint, history of present illness, past medical history, family medical history, review of symptoms and physical exam findings. The physician could include the diagnosis, lab findings, imaging findings and medical plan. With EMRs, the number of patients that can be seen in the same time frame can be 20, 30 or 40% lower than with paper charting with less accurate charting. I am unaware of any EMR that has increased the speed in which physicians can see and treat patients with accurate documentation. I am not aware of any improvement of care that has resulted from using EMRs. EMRs seemed designed more to meet coding and billing purposes as opposed to improving quality of care, benefitting the patient, or benefitting the treating physician. Because of the EMRs design, charting ends up being confusing and often contradictory. Many who use them simply "click" boxes without paying attention or understanding what they are charting making them inaccurate and defeating the accuracy and usefulness of EHRs. It has been reported that a physician must make over 1000-1500 clicks in order to complete EMRs in a single 12-hour shift. One could make the argument that this is bad for medicine and patient care. Physicians spend much more time with charting and other "paperwork" and less quality time with patients, up to 3 times more. It should do the opposite. Because EHRs take away from patient time and can make physician productivity decrease, many patients and physician have been hurt since their implementation. Intuitively this means that healthcare has taken another wrong turn and just another sign that our current healthcare system ignores common sense and what is best for patients.

One could make the argument that EHRs contribute to negligent, or fraudulent, charting

Some physicians and NPPs often document conflicting information within the same chart because they are so busy clicking on the various "boxes" that are required for billing purposes, that they do not even realize what they are charting. One could make the argument that the EHRs have contributed to negligent, or fraudulent, charting. This is not good for patient care, places physicians and NPPs at risk and could increase the costs of healthcare without improving care. EMRs have the potential to help physicians be more efficient, improve charting, be able to spend more quality time with patients or see more patients. In order to do so, the developers of EMRs must make the EMRs smart and adapt to the way a physician thinks and practices medicine. It must be customizable to each individual user allowing them to practice as they ordinarily do and to be able to capture the experience in an easier and simpler manner.

With current EHRs, even the "newer ones" at the time of writing, the physician or other users must learn how to enter data in the EHR that is not natural or most conducive to the manner that a physician naturally thinks, interacts with a patient or practices medicine. It is as if the physician must learn a new language or practice medicine in a different manner that is foreign to them. This is one reason why EHRs slow physicians down and fail to achieve their purpose of improving accurate documentation or helping those who treat patients in real time, now and in the future. Many companies can design an EMR, but I am not aware of one that has been able to design one that makes it easier for physicians to use, easily customizable to each individual physician or NPP and improves physician productivity without sacrificing quality. All while still meeting regulatory and billing requirements. It seems that companies design systems and sell them to administrators without taking into consideration or giving enough emphasis on what is best for the patient or the physician caring for the patient. It seems to be what is best for the company that sells the EMR. So long as they are able to sell it and make money, they seem less concerned with listening to a physician who uses it or incorporating changes that will actually improve productivity that will enable the physician to spend more time with patients instead of charting. One would think that if EHR companies wanted to be more successful and hospitals wanted to encourage physicians to welcome EHRs and be able to use them to improve patient care and efficiency, EHRs would be designed with the end user in mind; the physician who takes care of the patient. Until administrators or other decision makers hold EMR vendors accountable and demand that the EMRs take into consideration common sense, what is best for patients and those who directly care for and treat patients, and force these vendors to make a product that actually improves care, things are unlikely to change. The EHR should be made to cater to whatever is best for the physician user, not what suites the hospital's billing department or what is easiest for the people who sell the EHR.

Telehealth

Technology has made great strides and helped man do so much more today than we were able to do not long ago. Technology can play a big role in a better healthcare system. I believe Telehealth is one such technology that is an important part of the solution to improving healthcare. It is a disruptive technology that will change medicine forever. Telehealth, the electronic transmission of audiovisual health information between a patient located at a "home" location and a provider located a different "distant" location, would be available in real time 24/7/365 to every patient. Telemedicine is not a new form of medicine. Telemedicine is the vehicle, tool or instrument that a physician or other NPP uses to practice their specialty in medicine or healthcare. It allows a physician to provide her services to a patient that is not in the same location. It is a vehicle that could exponentially increase the availability of specialists to patients across the country and globe. When I learned about this technology some years ago, I realized its potential. I became involved nationally and currently serve as the Chair of the American College of Emergency Physicians (ACEP) Telehealth Section (2018-2020). Telehealth offers:

- Immediacy of access
- Leveraging of resources i.e. one physician could provide care in multiple locations around the country and the world at the same time, or within seconds
- Convenience to patients
- Reduction or elimination of nosocomial infections
- High level care to rural and remote areas
- Care in disaster settings
- Protection to healthcare workers from radiation exposure in nuclear accidents
- Containing the spread of contagious diseases
- Protection to healthcare workers from highly contagious diseases i.e. viruses, bacteria, etc.
- Care in the biological setting i.e. warfare or other
- Sparing of safety equipment
- Care in the maritime and aviation setting
- Care to correctional facilities
- Care to those offshore
- Ability to care for soldiers in the battlefield
- Education and supervision of healthcare workers

- Almost anything one can imagine.

I encouraged my fellow emergency physicians, and all other physicians, to be engaged in telemedicine as it has so many applications in medicine and will be a major factor in medicine. We are only one major disaster, epidemic, pandemic or attack away from the world realizing how necessary and valuable telehealth is.

In March 2015, as far as I am aware, I was the first in the state of Louisiana to provide Tele-Emergency services to patients in an emergency department that had no physician in the ER. At the time, I was the medical director of a couple ERs, one a relatively busy 55,000 patient visits per year ER and another smaller ER with approximately 15,000 patient visits per year. It took some convincing of the administrator and medical staff, but I was able to get the OK and implement a pilot study at the smaller ER. We wanted to test the effectiveness of having a non-physician provider (physician assistant) stationed in the ER with back-up by an emergency medicine residency trained board certified physician via telemedicine vs. the typical staffing at that ER that used physicians who were not board certified in emergency medicine. All patients in the pilot study were seen by the emergency physician via telemedicine. The pilot study report demonstrated that during the pilot study period:

- An improvement in quality metrics
- Shorter wait times from the time a patient arrives in the ER until they are placed in an exam room ("door to room time")
- Shorter wait times from the time a patient arrives in the ER until they are seen by the NPP ("door to doc time")
- Shorter wait times from the time a patient is placed in an exam room until they are seen by a NPP ("room to doc time")
- Shorter total time in the ER, from arrival to discharge or admission ("length of stay")
- Less use of expensive and potentially harmful radiological testing. During the pilot, patients seen and treated via telemedicine on average had 0.83 images per patient and 0.17

CT scans per patient compared to patients seen using the non-telemedicine traditional ER visit using non-emergency physicians who averaged 1.35 (>60% more) images per patient and 0.31 (>80% more) CT scans per patient.

- Higher patient satisfaction

Telehealth allows for any physician or NPP involved in the patient's care team, from physician to nurse practitioner to physician assistant to dietician to social worker etc., to be able to interact with the patient at any time of day by appointment or even within minutes if required. Such a system would allow multiple physician and non-physician providers, if needed in the patient's health, to have "Health Rounds," a conference call simultaneously. Such calls that involve a "multi-disciplinary team" with experts in whatever is necessary for a particular patient that might include a combination of any of the following: PCP, surgeon, endocrinologist, neurologist, pulmonologist, etc., dietician, physical or occupational therapist, social worker, HC, insurance representative, nurse, respiratory therapist, wound care specialist, etc. This allows those involved in the health of a patient to discuss simultaneously and in real time like rounds that occur in an organized and efficient hospital intensive care unit (ICU) when dealing with patient with complex conditions.

This would increase efficiency by having everyone on a patient's care team discuss any plan in real time and negate the need to have additional calls and repeat what was previously discussed by others. It could avoid confusion and misunderstandings by the patient or members of the health care team. It would allow any provider who might have a concern with any plan to bring it up in real time. This would avoid something being done that may not be the best action for a patient and then having to notify everyone else in the treatment group about the need to change. If it is done in real time, this preventable and time consumer chore, which could also be detrimental to the patient's care, could be avoided altogether. Technology and various entrepreneurial advancements would include Telehealth, home delivery of food, medication and most any other medical supply or service to the patient whenever and wherever it is most convenient and beneficial to the patient.

It is interesting how some things go full circle. An example of this is the "House Call." This was once commonplace. Decades ago, when someone was ill, physicians would go to their home to care for them. When a doctor went to a person's home, this was known as a house call. Whether it was out of kindness, because customer service mattered, because competition was greater and doctors were trying to expand their practices or because doctors cared more back then and were willing to do what was best for their patients, even if it was not what was best for the doctor, doctors commonly made house calls. This was common prior to 1970 and even continued into the 1970s but seemed to fade away and has become almost, if not completely, extinct. Practices became busier and often moved away from residential areas to medical complexes, the insurance industry became more developed, dominant and demanding, and many regulations were put in place. Safety became a concern. It seemed one of the best and most convenient things about healthcare for patients was taken away from patients. Those who remember the time when house calls were regularly made, might have even had a physician come to their home to treat them during their time of need, and remember how nice it was not to have to move, get dressed, get into a car and travel in pain or feeling sick, having to wait in a doctor's office or emergency department's waiting room before being seen, may miss the house call. Unfortunately, the house call all but disappeared. Some high-end concierge practices still offer the service to those willing to pay for the convenience, but this is the exception, not the rule.

With available technology, the House Call can become a common service again

Unfortunately, most people are unable to afford or justify the cost of concierge medicine...until now. With the advancements of technology, newer equipment and better telecommunication services and infrastructure, the house call is no longer only available to those who have significant means. We call this Telehealth. While it is not exactly the same, Telehealth can offer many of the conveniences and advantages of the house call; it allows quality care in your home or other location, without you having to move to a distant location to see the doctor. The physician is brought to you "virtually." So, in a sense, Telehealth has brought back the much-loved house call. The house call that almost went extinct because of how the healthcare industry "matured." The house call that almost went extinct because the healthcare industry seemed to ignore what the patient wants or prefers. The house call has come full circle and is making a comeback because technology has made Telehealth possible. It is not surprising how well received telehealth is with patients. Many patients prefer telehealth to an in-person physician visit. Is this because patients do not like in-person visits or patients prefer the convenience of having the visit whenever and wherever the patients want. It is unclear if patients would prefer a telehealth visit to an in-person house call visit.

Dr. HouseCall MD® (drhousecallmd.com) offers a hybrid of telehealth and an in-person experience

While in residency training in Orlando, I made house calls to patients visiting Walt Disney World from out of town. Even though I did not directly work for Disney, many referred to me as the "Disney Doctor." This experience made me realize how much people still value having a doctor come to them as opposed to having to go to an emergency room or urgent care center. I have been involved with Telehealth for some years. It hit me that I could merge the two. I named it Dr. HouseCall MD® (drhousecallmd.com). With this service, a hybrid of telehealth and an in-person experience is offered. A service that provides in-person visits at home and uses telehealth to deliver a board certified specialist to the patient to take a complaint focused history, perform an exam, develop a differential diagnosis, plan an action plan and oversee care and treatment to the patient in the patient's home. Telehealth can take place in the most-simple manner by a person using a smart phone APP or other Health Information Privacy and Accountability Act (HIPAA) compliant platform in their home, or just about any other location, to connect to a physician in a remote location to provide the physician's services. It can also be as advanced or involved as specially trained health personnel, known as a Mobile Medical Team (MMT), being sent to the patient, in-person and onsite in the patient's home or other location, with the backup of a physician specialist via telehealth as is the case with the Dr. HouseCall MD's house call business model. The remotely located board certified physician specialist can see the patient, talk to the patient, develop differential diagnoses, create a treatment plan and oversee care for the patient. With added peripherals, the remote physician specialist can listen to the patient's heart and lung sounds, examine the patients ears, nose, eyes, throat or other body part needed in a manner similar to what the physician could do if the physician is at the patient's bedside or the physician and patient are having a traditional in-person interaction. This can all be done in the comfort and familiar environment of one's home. In a sense, DrHouseCallMD.com can bring the ER to you, instead of you having to go to the ER.

Tele-Hospitals are possible. Such an entity would allow a person to be able to obtain many of the same benefits that one might get from going to a hospital. A way of looking at a Tele-Hospital is like this. Just as Dr. HouseCall MD can bring the ER to you, Tele-Hospital can bring the hospital to you. Just as you might go to the emergency room for a symptom, illness or injury, and be seen by an emergency physician (EP) who would evaluate and treat you, a Tele-Hospital could do the same. You could connect via smart phone or other device that has equipment that could help transmit medical information i.e. camera, stethoscope, otoscope, etc., and be evaluated by an emergency physician (EP). If your complaint could be managed just through simple telehealth, that is where the call/connection would end. If medications were needed, the telehealth EP would electronically prescribe them and send to the patient's preferred pharmacy and you could pick them up or they could be delivered to your door. If someone has a laceration or other complaint that might need hands on care, treatment or a procedure performed, a Mobile Medical Team (MMT) with special training could be summoned and sent to the patient's home such as is the case with the DrHouseCallMD.com Model.

Once onsite, the procedure could be performed by the medical team under the supervision of the board-certified emergency physician. Any of these services that are done or overseen by an emergency specialist would be considered a Tele-Emergency visit.

Should the EP determine that you need the services of a specialist i.e. cardiologist, neurologist, pediatrician, GI, etc., the appropriate specialist could be summoned to participate on the Telehealth call and participate in the patient's care. This is how an EP in the traditional ER might consult a specialist to come see a patient in the ER. Any services requiring a specialist beyond the emergency specialist would require the EP consulting that specialist just as is done when you go to the ER. A Tele-Hospital allows the Tele-Emergency Specialist to consult other Tele-Specialists. The benefit of telehealth is that this could all be done while the patient is in the comfort of his or her home. Tele-Hospitals have the potential to bring the hospital and all of its specialists to your home. Care being provided in the patient's home, and outside of the hospital, is the future of medicine and healthcare. By not having to go to the hospital, patients avoid 100% of the nosocomial infections i.e. Methicillin-resistant Staphylococcus aureus (MRSA), Clostridium difficile (C. diff), Coronavirus (COVID-19), Influenza, etc. Patients suffering from dementia who may get disoriented because of unfamiliar surroundings or environments could avoid this disorientation and the complications that sometimes can be associated with it.

Patients do not have to arrange for expensive or inconvenient transportation or incur the potential pain associated with movement for some conditions. They can be seen by specialists that are otherwise not available to them in their area. For example, if there is a particular expert in endocrinology at the Mayo clinic in Minnesota, an expert neurologist in Houston and an expert pancreatic oncology surgeon in Baltimore, a patient could potentially "see" and receive treatment from each of them in the same day without ever having to leave the patient's home in Kentucky, California, Texas, New York, Florida, Alaska, Hawaii, Paris, London, Sydney, Tokyo or anywhere else. When one thinks about it, telehealth has opened so many doors and offers so many opportunities not before possible, for us to make healthcare better than ever.

Although slow to come around, the government is starting to see the light and make some steps in the right direction to help allow telehealth to reach its full potential. In 2019, the Centers for Medicare and Medicaid Services (CMS) initiated a program known as ET3. "Emergency Triage, Treat and Transport (ET3) is a voluntary, five-year payment model that will provide greater flexibility to ambulance care teams to address emergency health care needs of Medicare beneficiaries following a 911 call."[114] Perhaps its intention is to reduce unnecessary ambulance transports to the ER and reduce unnecessary expensive emergency room visits. Perhaps it is to encourage more appropriate use of the Emergency Medical Services (EMS) and emergency department services. When EMS is called, the EMS personnel will no longer necessarily be required to transport everyone to the emergency department as they may presently be required to do. The patient can be evaluated by an emergency physician via telehealth to determine:

- If the patient has an emergency and requires transportation to the emergency department
- If the patient can be evaluated and determined to not have anything requiring immediate treatment and be referred to a lower cost physician or healthcare entity such as an urgent care or PCP's office
- If the EP can evaluate the patient and simply provide treatment via telehealth at the patient's home and not require any further treatment or transportation. If a patient does not have an

emergency but requires transportation, a friend can take the patient, or the patient can take a cab, Uber or Lyft.

In all cases, Medicare will pay for the service to evaluate and treat the patient at the patient's home. Before ET3, Medicare would not pay for care provided using telemedicine at a patient's home. It is my understanding that to encourage EMS to participate in the ET3 pilot, the EMS will be paid the charge for ambulance transportation regardless of whether the patient is transported by ambulance or not. It is possible that Medicare did this to encourage EMS providers to participate. If Medicare only paid EMS providers when patients were actually transported and not pay them if the patient was instructed to call a cab or have a friend drive them, EMS providers may be unwilling to participate in the ET3 pilot program or somehow find a reason to transport patients to the emergency department which would allow them to bill and collect payment for the transport. While there may be some Emergency Medical Treatment and Labor Act (EMTALA) and other concerns, if planned, implemented and done properly, ET3 has the potential of removing lots of waste and still provide quality care at a much lower cost. In addition, it should reduce the time EMS personnel are tied up transporting non-emergency patients and free them up for other calls that may be life threatening and require emergent transportation. It should also reduce the burden of overcrowded ERs allowing more serious ER patients to receive care sooner and allowing emergency staff more time to spend with and care for more serious patients. To the credit of Medicare leaders, they realize that the current system is broken and are looking for ways to improve at least one part of the broken system. It is unfortunate that private payers have not done a better job or taken the lead in such efforts. Perhaps they want to wait and see how Medicare's ET3 project works out before changing their reimbursement model.

Interestingly, Medicare was vague on compensation to the EP who would participate in the ET3 program It is reported that there would be compensation for the physician but I am not aware if they will be paying the same as they would be paid had they seen the patient in the ER. It would only be fair. If EMS is being paid the full amount whether or not they provide transport, it only seems fair to pay the EP for their service since they are providing it each and every time. I asked CMS to do so. Furthermore, I asked the Center for Medicare and Medicaid Services (CMS) and government officials to:

- Allow all patients, regardless of where they are located, to have the choice of being treated via Telemedicine i.e. at home, work, health facility, etc.
- Require payers i.e. insurers, to allow any licensed physician to provide the services
- Require payers to pay the same amount as they would if the service were provided in person (parity)

Hopefully, these common-sense ideas will be implemented into CMS policy and adopted by all private insurers and payers and become the standard. If done, Telehealth will become the norm as it is can be a superior form of care. Time will tell.

In late 2019, SARS-nCoV-2, also called COVID-19 or Coronavirus 19, emerged in Wuhan China and by March 2020 became a worldwide pandemic. The United States was not spared. Given the significance of the virus, how it had quickly spread, the manner that it was reported to the American public, particularly by the media, there was a panic. The public rushed retail stores and "cleared the shelves" of disinfectant wipes, disinfectant sprays, liquid bleach, toilet paper, hand sanitizers and other items. Water and many food products were hoarded by the public. According to the CDC update on March 13, 2020, the total number of cases of COVID-19 in the United States was 1629 and the death toll 41.[115]

I expect the number of people to test positive to rise dramatically once testing becomes more widespread. Sadly, the number of deaths caused by the virus is will likely rise. If I had to guess the number of deaths directly related to SARS-nCoV-2, I would say it will be comparable to a bad flu season from Influenza or even pass it. Of course, the "official number" could be even higher if deaths are blamed on COVID-19 for anyone who dies even if the actual cause was from something else but that person happened to have a positive test or symptoms that could have been consistent with COVID-19. I imagine that the vast majority of people have little or no symptoms so if someone dies in a motor vehicle accident, heart attack, suicide or drug overdose that tests positive, will that person be counted as a COVID-19 death or more accurately from the most likely cause of death? Unfortunately, if one has an agenda, they can manipulate the numbers to support that agenda. What is the saying? "Figures don't lie but liars figure?" We must be careful not to believe what anyone says until we look at things and interpret the data in an unbiased manner that is not agenda driven.

One can debate how the Coronavirus pandemic was handled and if blame should be assigned. I already see many things that could have been done better but I do not believe being critical during a crisis is helpful to the country. There will be plenty of time to do that later. Right now, I believe we should rally around our elected officials and work together to fight our common enemy: the virus that is causing illness and death of our fellow Americans and world inhabitants.

The reason I mention the COVID-19 pandemic is to point out one of the many valuable aspects of telehealth that I have advocated as an individual, and later as the ACEP's Telehealth Section Chair that became quite apparent during the national emergency that was declared in March 2020, Telehealth avoids unnecessarily exposing patients and healthcare workers. Telehealth allows physicians to evaluate patients at their home or any other location that possesses adequate telecommunication capabilities. One of the biggest concerns with COVID-19, and other contagious illnesses, is that it can spread by interacting with others. During the COVID-19 pandemic, the public was encouraged to stay at home and not come to the hospital or ER to be checked unless their condition was serious. These recommendations were meant to decrease the chance of spreading the illness to others, particularly those who are most at risk such as the elderly or those with significant underlying diseases. Telemedicine was mentioned quite frequently, by numerous politicians, as an effective and valuable way to provide medical attention without putting physicians or other health care providers at risk or unnecessarily exposing others to the illness. Even the President of the United States touted telemedicine and signed into law the Coronavirus legislation on March 6, 2020 that expands the use of telemedicine in outbreak areas.[116] Numerous states also eased the rules for the practice of telemedicine. During the emergency, Texas Governor Greg Abbott asked insurance companies to waive the costs associated with testing and telemedicine visits associated with the diagnosis of Coronavirus.[117] Governor Andrew Cuomo of New York required insurance companies to waive the co-pay on all tele-health visits.[118] Finally, government may be getting it and realizing the potential of telemedicine that drew me to it many years ago.

I have long advocated for the expansion of telemedicine and continue to do so as Chair of the Telehealth Section. I encouraged government and private payers to reimburse for telemedicine because I realized the obvious advantages to patients long before the Wuhan Flu (SARS-nCoV-2) caused illness and death in the United States. It just made sense. Other than being able to provide convenient and quality care to the patient in their home, it prevents the spread of infections and nosocomial infections i.e. infections that people get from being in the hospital or other health care facilities. If someone is treated in their home, not the ER or hospital, they cannot get a nosocomial infection. They also cannot expose others who are located at a different location. It was refreshing to see that finally the leaders of our country saw benefits of telemedicine that I have been championing for so long.

History will show whether shelter-in-place for so many and shutting down the economy for so long were the wisest decisions

It is unfortunate that the American way of life and economy were so severely disrupted and are likely to suffer even more if the shutdown continues. While I can only assume it was done with good intention, I am not sure that history will show that shelter-in-place for so many and shutting down the economy was the wisest decision. Some will argue that it was. Human life is more important than money or the American economy or way of life.

Others will argue that the decision to declare an emergency, shut down the economy and have people remain in their homes and not be able to attend church, see loved ones, attend funerals or be with one's loved one(s) in their last moments of life was not the best decision. They will add that we may never be sure that doing so actually will save lives in the long run and could cause more deaths and harm than it prevents. If one considers the suffering and loss of life that result from job loss, poverty, hunger, depression, suicide, domestic and child abuse, alcohol and drug abuse and resulting overdoses that may result from the shutting down the economy and the shelter in place orders, we may have caused more deaths and suffering than had we allowed people to continue to work. In addition, there are the ethical issues, possible governmental overreach and the individual, civil and constitutional rights that may have been violated.

Of course, common sense things as hand washing that should have always been done, and masks would have been reasonable as they can protect and help but still allow the economy to continue to support our way of life. It also would have saved our country trillions upon trillions of dollars that were spent that will add significantly to our national debt, cause more pain in the future to many, and will have to be paid down if we ever want to be fiscally responsible. I understand the reasoning, but history may show the spending may not have been needed if the shutdown was not needed. History may one day tell us if the shutdown caused more death and suffering than allowing things to continue as we typically do during a flu season but perhaps using more frequent hand washing, wearing masks, sheltering in place for only those most vulnerable and discouraging large gatherings. It is complicated because it is more than a simple medical matter, it also involves economics, ethics, individual rights, etc. and these factors must be considered. But further discussion is better suited for another time or another book.

In addition to telehealth, technology may include the use of more recent services such as "futuristic" delivery systems such as robots, drones or other things that may not have even been implemented, invented, or created as of this writing. Be it the home, the nursing home, the patient's place of business or any other location, technology allows us to "transport" the service, medication, or meal to the patient. Same goes for other services, or other future services, that do not even yet exist or that we are aware. The point is a great healthcare system is patient obsessed©. Whatever is best for the patient is the goal. A great healthcare system empowers those within healthcare to do whatever in reasonable that must be done, in order to achieve what is best for the patient and/or public. If it does not yet exist, a great healthcare, or benevolent capitalistic, system will figure out a way to develop it. Unlike the current healthcare system that seems to focus around the convenience or demands of the healthcare complex players, a great healthcare system goes out of its way to figure out a way to wow the patient by doing whatever is best for the patient and brings the best health to the patient. Satisfying the patient is not enough, we should impress them and try to exceed expectations every time. That is what people do who are committed to helping people, doing the right thing, and making healthcare the best it can possibly be.

No longer should a patient always have to make a trip to the doctor and incur all the inconveniences, stress, hassles and waiting involved. No longer should mildly ill people have to go to the hospital or physicians' offices to receive care or potentially infect health professionals or others. No longer should the patient have to make a trip to the pharmacy to drop off a prescription and wait for it to be filled or make another trip to come back and pick it up. No longer should a patient have to go to the grocery store to shop for the foods that their condition requires. This may sound like no big deal to some. What is the big deal? The big deal is that some people cannot walk. Some cannot drive. Some must depend on others for transportation. For some, it is painful to walk, or they may fall. Some may be too weak. Some may have weak immune systems and being exposed to people, let alone sick people in a doctor's waiting room, may cause a life-threatening infection. When a person is elderly, he may not be able to do some things that many take for granted. When someone is debilitated, they may not be able to do things that others take for granted. When someone is sick or injured, they are not at their best. They may simply not feel like going anywhere or it may be physically difficult to go anywhere. Technology makes it possible for the doctor to come "see" the patient virtually, examine, diagnose and treat them. Technology allows for prescriptions to be electronically sent to a pharmacy and delivered to the patient's front door. Technology allows food meeting your dietary requirements, to be delivered to your door. All without you ever leaving the comfort, security and safety of your home or bed.

Digital health and artificial or augmented intelligence (AI), will also play a role. We will use AI to represent both artificial and augmented intelligence. As AI advances, it will be able to take on a greater role and help provide better healthcare. Interestingly, AI has the advantage in that it "learns" as it goes and becomes better and better with time. Sounds like people. Doctors learn in medical school and with experience, often seem to get better and better. Unlike people who can forget what they have learned, get older and retire, or eventually die off, AI never dies. It does not forget and will only learn more and improve itself. Instead of having to train a new radiologist or dermatologist, AI with time will be able to read any X-ray or scan and recognize any skin condition or disease and will only get more and more accurate as it has more data that it has reviewed. AI can have the equivalent "experience" of hundreds or thousands of doctors. There is already data emerging showing the promise of AI. "Google's artificial intelligence development has reached a milestone in lung cancer imaging and prediction, with a CT scan model being able to diagnose cases as well as or better than a group of six radiologists."[119] The future is promising. Whether or not people are ever eliminated from providing healthcare to you or the public is not the point or necessarily the goal of AI in my opinion, it is whether AI can help make our healthcare system better. I believe if used responsibly, it will.

Chapter 13 Talking Points:

- Instead of improving quality and efficiency, electronic medical records seem more focused on billing and collection and can be detrimental to quality care best use of time.
- Telehealth can provide safe, convenient, and affordable care, anytime and anyplace to patients by any physician located anywhere.
- Telemedicine allows the ER, hospital or doctor to be brought to the patient's home. DrHouseCallMD.com is a leader in pioneering this "revolution" in healthcare. Not only does
- Dr. HouseCall MD does not only simple telemedicine, but also will offer Mobile Medical Teams to come to a patient's home to provide IV fluids and medications, provide other treatments and perform procedures in the comfort of one's home
- Technology and Augmented Intelligence are showing promise and may improve healthcare beyond what can be done by humans
- Telehealth offers the advantage of avoiding exposure to nosocomial infections associated with hospitals and other dangerous exposures i.e. radiation, SARS-nCoV-2 a.k.a. Wuhan Flu, Coronavirus, COVID-19, Influenza

Chapter Fourteen:
MEDICARE FOR ALL

When I set upon the journey to write *Make Healthcare Great Again*, it was not my intention to include "Medicare for All" (MFA). However, I decided to include a brief discussion in response to the many inquiries I received from others; it seems to be important to many people. MFA has come up a lot in the current 2019-2020 presidential political campaign and seems to have many concerned and talking about it. As I was writing, many asked me about MFA. Is it a good idea? Would it save money? Would it change Medicare as it exists today? Would it affect doctors, hospitals, and patients? Would it make things better? Would it make things worse?

MFA has been suggested by some as a means improve our healthcare system, specifically the insurance coverage that will pay for our healthcare. This idea has been proposed as a solution to the private insurance dominated healthcare that is prevalent in the United States. Bernie Sanders, the US Senator, and democratic presidential candidate from Vermont, advocated for MFA. Others have promoted the idea and have come up with various versions of what MFA should "look like." While I can only assume that their intentions are good, it is my opinion that it would be more harmful to America's healthcare and its people than any potential benefits.

It is my understanding that MFA would apply to everyone. 100% of the population would have it. There is some debate as to whether there would still be private insurance as an option, but I guess it depends on the candidate and the political climate as candidates tend to change their views and opinions depending on polling and other factors.

Assuming everyone would be required to have Medicare and we would do away with private insurance, it would be a problem. This would essentially dictate to Americans what insurance they have. Put another way, Americans would not have a choice. This alone should be reason enough to be weary of MFA. I advocate the right to choose. Americans do not like not having choice. In this country, we have come to expect freedom and with freedom comes choice. So, from a pure principal point of view, Medicare for All is bad. While some may call it innovative, it seems to be neither innovative nor good for the public.

MFA, if modeled after Medicare, is destined for failure. Most people may not realize this, but Medicare does not cover the costs of doing business for many hospitals and physicians. Private insurers subsidize the losses, of hospitals and physician staffing companies that accept Medicare patients and allow hospitals, physicians and other NPPs to survive financially. Currently, there are many physicians, particularly specialists that do not currently accept Medicare as payments for this reason. Even some hospitals don't accept Medicare. One may wonder why? It is because the amount that Medicare reimburses for the care does not justify the work, time, costs, regulatory requirements and liability involved with seeing and treating Medicare patients. According to information presented by the CEO of one of the largest physician staffing companies in the country during the ACEP Leadership and Advocacy Conference in Washington DC in 2019, for each dollar of actual provider compensation Medicare only pays 97%.[120] Put another way, Medicare does not even cover the costs of providing care to Medicare patients. Many hospital administrators might tell you that hospitals do not make money on Medicare patients. I have heard this on numerous occasions. So, if we instituted MFA and all other things stayed the same, based on this information, all physician staffing companies would go out of business. Companies and hospitals cannot and do not want to lose money, they do not want to break even; they want to make money, profits. Medicaid is even worse. Medicaid only pays 50% of the actual physician compensation. Uninsured patients only pay 23% of actual physician costs. And there would no longer be the profitable private insurance that could subsidize any losses from Medicare patients.

Medicare for ALL will cost $30+ trillion dollars in 10 years, which is more than America's total debt accumulated between 1776 and 2020

The thought of eliminating private health insurance and converting over to Medicare to solve all our problems is ridiculous. Medicare would have to cover so many more people than they currently do who are not able to or will not pay into Medicare. Costs of Medicare will drastically increase. Where would the subsidy come from? Higher taxes? Higher withholdings from paychecks? MFA would cause the Medicare program to go bankrupt and collapse or it would have to significantly change. Perhaps, the idea is to raise taxes or reduce Medicare services in order to make the numbers work. Perhaps, the numbers will not work regardless. Spending an extra $30+ trillion dollars in 10 years, which is more than America's total debt it has accumulated in its entire existence since 1776, is concerning and cause for worry. This is the important information that the candidates and advocates for MFA fail to discuss or explain well. Wonder why?

If the government were to have MFA, which would be the equivalent of a health insurance monopoly, it is hard to imagine that it would be effective, efficient or promote what is best for the public. Historically monopolies are not considered good for the public. Standard oil was a huge energy company owned by John Rockefeller. The government forced it to break up because the government determined that monopolies were "not in the best interest of the public" or our country. So, why should the public suddenly tolerate or want a health payer monopoly run by the government, an entity known for inefficiencies, waste and sometimes corruption?

MFA would likely cause a decline in the quality of medical treatment or decrease access to care. If government pays less, it is very possible the capable and qualified people who might go into medicine may instead choose to pursue other professions where they can earn a better living for themselves and provide a better life for their families. MFA may cause a situation where everyone may be insured but the sick may not be able to receive care without delays in treatment or even denial of care altogether. Consider the Veteran's Administration (VA). This is a government run health program for veterans. Many veterans are made to wait weeks or months for appointments or to receive treatment that privately insured patients can get immediately or within days. I have heard stories that in England, people with hip fractures are sent home to await needed hip surgeries which could be weeks or months, whereas in the United States such patients currently have the surgery the same or next day. Same goes for people requiring coronary artery bypass graft surgery (CABG) or "heart bypass" surgery. Outside the United States, if someone is discovered to require a CABG, they may be sent home with medications and must wait days, weeks or months for the surgery. Sometimes, these patients die at home from a heart attack while awaiting the necessary surgery. In the United States, such patients are often operated on the very day the surgery is discovered to be needed. Is this what we want for our country? This may be the consequences of Medicare for All.

Medicare for All would cost between $30 and $40 trillion over a decade dwarfing the estimated $940B cost of Obamacare over a decade[121]

What if the powers that be determine you do not qualify to have a needed procedure or surgery? Who will be the person or panel that determines what is needed or not? What will be your options if you are told no? Will you have a choice in what treatments you have? These are all things to consider before we trust government and abandon private insurance and personal choice. Of course, one should never say never but I am not sure I could ever support any policy, by any party, that eliminates the individual's ability to make choices for themselves. This is not a political issue. It is a health and freedom issue that affects us all regardless of political affiliation.

The ACA was supposed to lower premium costs. After the ACA became law, the cost of insurance premiums skyrocketed

It was not too long ago when the Affordable Care Act was passed. It was promised that the costs of healthcare would go down and if you liked your doctor, you could keep your doctor. Many will admit, perhaps even some of those who voted for the then new legislation, that neither of these two promises turned out not to be true. Many could no longer see the same doctors and the costs of health insurance rose considerably, as did deductibles. The public was told the ACA would lower premium costs. After the ACA became law, the cost of insurance premiums skyrocketed. The public has justifiably learned to be skeptical of political promises. There is at least one thing worse than the current broken healthcare system. It would be abandoning it for an even worse system. A system that takes away choice, makes accessing healthcare more difficult, may deny care, and costs so much more that it likely would bankrupt Medicare and potentially bankrupt the country. A bill released by Medicare for All Caucus co-chair Pramila Jayapal (D-WA) is estimated to cost taxpayers $28-$32 trillion dollars over a decade.[122] It is reported that Bernie Sanders stated that Medicare for All would cost between $30 and $40 trillion over a decade dwarfing the estimated $940B cost of Obamacare over a decade.[123] As expensive as many believe Obamacare was, Medicare for All makes it seem cheap.

During the June 26, 2019 democratic presidential debate, candidate John Delaney stated:

> "If you go to every hospital in this country and you ask them one question, which is, how would it have been for you last year if every one of your bills were paid at the Medicare rate? Every

single hospital administrator said they would close."[124]

While this may not be completely true for all hospitals, many hospitals and other health providers, stand to lose significant amounts of money if they are paid Medicare rates, which can be less than half what private insurers pay, for their services. Another article reports that Medicare for All could put most rural hospitals at "high risk" to close.[125]

While Medicare for All seems destined for failure, there is some good news. At least people are trying to come up with better ways to do things. That is a good thing. We need to come up with many ideas. We need to think them through, be critical about them. We must keep politics out of healthcare. Healthcare is important to the individual and to our country and should be taken very seriously. If an idea can withstand criticism and still seems to be a good idea that makes sense, morally, ethically and financially, then it may be worthy of being more seriously considered. If something makes sense, then we should consider trying it on a small scale. Do a pilot study designed by smart and politically unbiased people and see if it works. Objectively, set quality and cost measures before implementation and then analyze the outcomes and data after experimenting in a few locations. Ask people what they think. Get the opinions of the public who are affected by the pilot study. Get the objective, unbiased data and have trusted, unbiased intelligent people analyze the data, not politicians or politically influenced people. At that point, we can determine if it is a good thing or not, if it needs to be expanded or shut down or if it needs to be tweaked.

Why do we have to do it for every location in America and every American all at once? The ideas presented in this book are sound. Much thought has been put into them and I am happy to defend them. If they can't stand up to criticism and still seem to be good ideas from a care, morality, ethical and financial standpoint, we can tweak them or eliminate them. I am interested in helping people, not forcing people to do something and or taking away their right to choose. Even if the ideas I present withstand criticism and everyone thinks they are the answer that will fix everything, I still would not demand or expect every city in America to immediately implement them at the same time or that we should do away with every other option. That would be foolish and irresponsible. I say that and I am the guy who wrote the book. I do believe we should seriously consider these ideas, discuss them and perhaps roll them out to be tested.

It seems irresponsible for anyone who considers themselves a leader, especially someone who seeks to become President of our great country, to be ready and willing to take away the public's choice and change something that will affect everyone without first trying it out and making sure it make sense, works and is the best choice for the United States and its citizens. America and Americans are big on personal freedoms and choice. I believe people are not stupid. Some may be uneducated or not experts in healthcare, but they are not stupid. If something is so good, there is free flow of accurate information, there is a responsible free market, and people have freedom to choose, people will make the best decisions for themselves. Isn't that what we want? Isn't that the best option? So why not try various models and ideas and see what works best. People will pick what is best for them if we provide the proper setting, accurate and proper information and allow free choice. Give them incentives and disincentives. That is what makes sense. Not all ideas are going to work but diversification seems to give us a better chance of coming up with more options and better ideas that will work, and avoids risking putting "all our eggs in one basket" setting us up for a potential disaster. Just because something is a new idea, comes from someone we like or seems interesting does not make it good or better.

As a side note, it is my understanding that the big argument for passing the ACA was that 15% of the population was not insured. It is also my understanding that rates have increased significantly since the ACA was passed. In some cases, policy premiums have gone up over 100%. Many people were unhappy with the consequences of the ACA i.e. losing their doctor, higher rates and deductibles, etc. If 15% of the population did not have coverage and the intention of the ACA was to make sure everyone was insured, why not simply add a 17.65% insurance tax to all policies? This would result in enough money to simply buy the uninsured 15% health insurance, and the 85% with insurance could keep the insurance they had. The 85% would have to pay just 17-18% that would be enough to spay for the insurance of the 15% who were not insured. This way, the already insured would only pay a 17-18% premium tax instead of a 100% or higher premium for insurance as is the case with many. Maybe this is too simple of a way of looking at it? I am no politician, but this seems like it would have been the simplest, easiest and least expensive option and would have achieved the goal of 100% coverage. Other than the 17-18% premium tax, no one should have been worse off. Everyone who was already insured should have been able to keep their doctor and their insurance, and everyone who was uninsured should have been able to have similar priced insurance compared to those who were previously insured.

A physician's goal is to do no harm. This rule would have been a good one to follow for those who came up with the ACA. Do the most good as possible and the least amount of harm. Even with the large increases that occurred as a result of the ACA, sometimes over 100% higher, many people were not able to keep their doctors as they were promised, and millions of others remained uninsured. One can say the ACA failed in this regard. To make matters worse, many more have expensive insurance that they cannot afford to use because of the high deductibles that many have after the ACA was enacted. Yes, these people may have insurance but may be worse off than having no insurance at all. Is it possible more people have less "usable" insurance? My point is that government and politicians are notorious for not coming up with good solutions and telling the public things that turn out not to materialize. So, when someone says MFA will fix things, we must not be naïve and simply accept it as gospel. The saying "fool me once shame on you, fool me twice shame on me" seems fitting. I hope Americans are too smart to be fooled again when it comes to government fixing healthcare with MFA. It is quite possible it would fail and cause a disaster that we cannot recover from.

History shows that people and the private sector are innovative and good at coming up with solutions. This is part of what made our country so great. Our country has the environment to nurture innovation, allow the free market to work and reward people for taking chances. This may explain why our country is responsible for so many innovations and great things: mass produced automobile, electricity, aviation, railroads, personal computers, iPhone, vaccines, medical cures, etc. There is no one simple quick fix for the disaster of a healthcare system that we have worked ourselves into over the past few decades. One cannot expect to provide the same level of care to more people for the same cost simply by changing payers if nothing material changes. We must eliminate waste and be more efficient and effective. We must change certain things that will reduce the need for healthcare; reduce the demand. People must be healthier alleviating the need for expensive treatment. We must be innovative and allow competition to flourish not restrict it. Let the free market, and people's freedom to choose, determine the winners and losers. Government does not need to own and control our healthcare, instead they need to make sensible rules and guidelines for the private sector that encourages the free flow of accurate information for those within healthcare to do the right thing for the public. Create an environment that aligns the best interest of the public with the best interest of the insurer or other healthcare player in the healthcare complex and one will find that things somehow miraculously seem to work themselves out and improve. Making healthcare better for the public is not rocket science but instead it requires:

- Common sense
- Simple economics
- Good judgment
- Understanding people
- Asking why?
- Understanding why things are the way they are
- Asking why things are not another way?

- Ignoring what special interest groups, biased naysayers and lobbyists are trying to tell you
- Knowing what you want as the result
- Figuring out a way to get there
- Doing the right thing
- Providing accurate and necessary information to people
- Having effective incentives and disincentives
- Protecting an individual's right to choose
- Make everyone in healthcare accountable

While Medicare for All may be a great soundbite and seem reasonable to some, it scares me because I see the likely disaster that it would bring. That is why I decided to include this discussion because I wanted to point out some obvious downsides. There are much better options and one must be aware of just a few of the many MFA risks so they can realize it is not the solution that we need. I encourage you to do your own unbiased research. Hear both sides and look at the facts. Once you have accurate information, you can reach your own conclusion.

Chapter 14 Talking Points:

- MFA could essentially create a monopoly in health insurance, eliminating choice to the public
- MFA could decrease access to care, delay time to being seen or treated and possibly deny care all together
- Medicare For All (MFA) would cost an estimated 30-40 times more than the Affordable Care Act (ACA) a.k.a. Obamacare ($30-40 Trillion vs. $940 Billion over 10 years)
- Freedom and the right to choose is something that many cherish and do not want to give up
- Government officials have a history of making promises and statements that later turn out not to come to fruition i.e. ACA will lower the cost of healthcare and people will be able to keep their doctors
- People should do their own research and get the facts so they can make good informed decision

Edward Shaheen, M.D.

MAKE HEALTHCARE GREAT AGAIN

Chapter Fifteen:
CONCLUSION

"Don't complain, you have your health." Simple, yet very profound. This statement was what my mother often told me as a child to help me gain perspective when I would complain about something not being fair or right. It was intended to help me realize how incredibly lucky I was. Even though my mother's belief in how important and valuable one's health is played a big part in my decision to become a doctor, I did not understand how significant her words were early on. It was not until I became a physician and began to see people who were ill, injured, in pain, unable to care for themselves, without hope and suffering that I began to start to understand the weight of her amazingly wise and profound words.

To this day, I am amazed by how intelligent and insightful she was. She may have been born into poverty, had little to no formal education, but she was an intelligent, hard-working woman with great compassion, empathy, values, and an incredibly positive and insightful view of life. She understood what was important in life, the big picture. Basically, she got it. She instilled in all her children the value of one's health. With rare exception, the most valuable thing anyone could ever possess. You can have "nothing" but if you have your health, you are wealthy. To this day, whenever I examine or treat a patient, I often think of my mother, how important health was to her and try to incorporate the many values and humility she tried to instill in her children. Whenever a patient or family member is kind enough and compliments me on my bedside manner, care, kindness or desire to help or do the right thing, I cannot help but remember my mother and if time allows, let the patient know that whatever good I have, I owe it to my wonderful mom. She was amazing and I hope she can look down and smile and know she is still making a difference in people's lives. Even though I appreciate what she said so much more now than I did as a child, I realize so many people take their good health for granted. People tend to complain about all the things in life that they do not have and do not enjoy the blessing of the wealth they possess in the form of the good health they possess.

A long time ago, healthcare was "great." It may not have been perfect, but it was simple and easy to understand. It was reasonably priced. If someone had insurance, it often meant that should they become sick or injured, their biggest concern was trying to get better. They did not have to worry about expensive medical bills like today or getting surprise bills. The health insurance companies did not shift so much of the responsibility of the medical bills on the patient through deductibles, co-pays, co-insurance, pre-existing conditions, etc.

People could choose whatever doctor or hospital to use and insurance would cover it. There was not the same confusion or frustration with in-network and out-of-network doctors or non-physician providers. Often doctors would make house calls to a patient's home to care for them.

Decades ago, people seemed healthier. They seemed more responsible. They ate less processed foods, were not as obese as we are today, were less sedentary and seemed to be more physically active. Political correctness did not deter people from being honest and potentially helping others.

Things have changed considerable over the past few decades. Healthcare has become more "corporate." Many physicians and other types of practitioners provide services but many of their practices are owned or influenced by hospitals, insurers or large companies that are often driven by profits. It seems that much in healthcare seems more focused on those who stand to financially benefit from treating, or not treating, the sick and injured i.e. hospitals, CMGs, insurance companies, etc. as opposed to being focused on the actual patient who is sick or injured.

Healthcare has moved away from spending more time with patients and towards ordering more expensive and sometimes unnecessary or harmful tests on patients. Healthcare costs have become a much greater percentage of our country's expenses, having increased at a rate far outpacing wages earned or inflation. Healthcare expenses are often a cause of financial stress, can easily wipe out a family's savings and is often a cause of debt or bankruptcy.

Can we make healthcare great again? I believe we can. Healthcare is complex but does not have to be complicated. The simpler we make healthcare:

- The more people will likely understand it
- The more people will be empowered
- The more likely people will make better decisions
- The more likely the public will benefit

Healthcare includes everyone and all entities that can affect or influence one's health. The healthcare complex includes everyone, actual human beings, and non-human entities, in healthcare except for the patient. Put into a mathematical equation: (Healthcare System - Patient = Healthcare Complex)

When discussing the many players in healthcare, I intentionally tried to present things from a patient's perspective as often as possible and discussed many of the reasons why the healthcare complex may behave the way it does. I also presented many possible solutions that could improve how many players in the healthcare complex could improve the services they provide and improve the care and service to patients. I have shown how the public is often kept in the dark by many in the healthcare complex. This interferes with a person's ability to make the best-informed decisions or the best decisions for themselves or their loved ones.

We must be creative and innovative, use our broad base of knowledge, good judgment and common sense and do what is best for the patient, the public and society. Making mistakes is not the end of the world; it is often the first step to improvement. So long as we recognize and learn from them, make the necessary adjustments, and continually improve. I discussed different ways to transform the insurance industry into having more incentive to do what is best for the patient, including the Direct Care Organization model. I discussed a way for the public to obtain information, in a simple, easy, and anonymous manner, so that people can make better informed healthcare decisions. We introduced the Healthy Mart concept to make it easier to shop for healthier food and food particular to one's specific diagnosis or needs i.e. D-meals. I discussed telemedicine and telehealth, how it is allows us to bring care to the patient, like the old days when the doctor would make a house call i.e. DrHouseCallMD.com

We must be realistic. We should not make assumptions. We must realize that healthcare not only consists of highly educated individuals, technological advancement, specialized equipment, specialists, special medications etc. but also the very simple and basic things such as a person's living conditions, whether or not they have shelter, clean water, heating or air conditioning, sanitation, electrical service, the ability to afford medication, food or other necessities, access to transportation, the ability to read and other things that if taken for granted interfere with one's ability to be healthy. While we must embrace technology and intelligently incorporate it into healthcare, we must understand that it does not replace or substitute for kindness, empathy, respect, humility, compassion and other important human values that are so important to quality healthcare and treating the person, not just the patient.

A very fundamental part of any great healthcare system is that the patient has choices to make great healthcare decisions for themselves. This includes choices on the proper diet, housing or shelter, lifestyle, and treatment if it is necessary. The patient must be informed, engaged, protected and capable of making good choices. Ultimately, the patient, or patient's guardian, should be the one who makes the final healthcare decision. All players in healthcare should be transparent. I discussed Price/Quality Disclosures, Medical and Medication Menus as simple, yet effective methods to improve transparency and make getting useful information, such as quality scoring and pricing, to patients and the public. I discussed other innovative or novel concepts as Healthy Marts, Diagnosis or "D" Meals, Policy Weakness Disclosures, Highlight Consent Forms, Telehealth, Tele-Hospitals, Mobile Medical Teams, Direct Care Organizations and Health Consultants or Medical Managers amongst others, as ways to help make things simpler and easier to understand and to enable people to eat properly, understand the quality of the care that is available or they are receiving; understand the price of the healthcare that is available or they are getting and perhaps even more importantly, the actual cost that the patient will be responsible for paying; and to help the patient understand and manage their healthcare with an "expert" or "consultant" i.e. Health Agent or Consultant, etc. that is familiar with the particulars of each patient.

I discussed the important role the patient and public have in healthcare. They have the final say as they are the patient. Patients are also consumers and can exert their power as selective consumers on suppliers of healthcare services so long as they have free choice. A well-informed patient is better equipped to make better decisions, find better prices, find higher quality services, negotiate better prices for goods and services and live healthier lives. In addition, they can influence and pressure government representative to represent their needs and demands. People have the ultimate power; we have our vote to cast in our free elections within our democratic republic. We have the power to fire our current elected representatives in the next election when their current term expires.

"Medicare for All" as discussed may sound reasonable until we understand what it really means and the many downsides to it that could worsen quality, decrease access to healthcare, deny care, eliminate the individual's choice and potentially bankrupt Medicare and the entire country.

I discussed the various players within healthcare and how each play a role in healthcare. Both the good and the not so good aspects of various players were discussed. There seems to be a common theme that keeps coming up. Many in the healthcare complex seem more focused on themselves as opposed to the patient. Often, this is to the detriment of the patient in the following ways:

- Lack of complete and accurate information
- Less access to healthcare
- Delays in receiving necessary testing or procedures
- Unnecessary tests and procedures being performed
- Higher healthcare costs
- Poorer health

Healthcare is important to the individual and all of us as a society. If we want to make healthcare great again, the following must occur:

- The healthcare complex needs to be patient obsessed©
- All players within the healthcare complex must align what is best for themselves with what is best for the public
- The healthcare complex must first do what is best for the patient, and a very close second, do what is best for those who take care of the patients
- People should be free to choose what is best for themselves and for those for whom they are responsible
- There needs to be consequences to every decision we make-good and bad
- There needs to be accurate and easy to understand information so the public can make better informed decisions-keep it simple
- There should be incentives and disincentives to encourage better choices that lead to better health and to discourage bad decisions that could lead to poor health
- Everyone must be responsible for themselves and must be held accountable for their choices, decisions, and actions

Competition, with few exceptions, is good and should be nurtured and encouraged. Usually, the more choices people have, the better it is for society; the better the quality may be and the less expensive the good or service will be. There needs to be incentives and disincentives to help align everyone in healthcare towards great healthcare. Financial incentives and profits, while not the only incentive and traditionally believed by many to be inherently bad, are not. If used properly, they can be quite effective and beneficial to the patient and the public.

By aligning all players in the healthcare space with what is best for the public, many costly monitoring programs, wastefulness, and inefficient processes almost magically disappear. The healthcare players start to do the right thing without having to be heavily monitored or supervised. They supervise themselves to be compliant because it is in their best interest and happens to be in the best interest of the patient and society. This concept is fundamental to having a successful and great healthcare system that works.

When bad choices or decisions are made, there must be consequences, regardless of whom makes them. Whether patients, insurers, hospitals or any other player in healthcare, everyone must be held accountable. We can no longer excuse bad decisions and reward or encourage the "victim mentality." We must protect the public's right to choose and empower people to do the right thing and make the correct choices. The current healthcare system is broken and needs to be fixed or replaced altogether. This is not a political position, it is fact. We must stop trying to be so politically correct at the expense of being honest and do things that will result in better health. We can no longer just try and reward the attempt or an intention or enable those who make poor choices. We must achieve and reward desired results. This will help assure that the individual and society ultimately will be better off.

If we can make changes and do the things discussed in, *Make Healthcare Great Again*:

- We will **make healthcare simpler to understand**
- We will **make healthcare easier to access**
- We will **make healthcare have more options for the public**

- We will **make healthcare patients be better informed**
- We will **make healthcare patients more empowered**
- We will **make healthcare more affordable**
- We will **make healthcare patients healthier** and,

WE WILL **MAKE HEALTHCARE GREAT AGAIN!**

GLOSSARY

A.k.a.-abbreviation for "also known as"

ACA-abbreviation for the Affordable Care Act, which is more accurately named the Patient Protection and Affordable Care Act. See Patient Protection and Affordable Care Act.

Advanced Practice Practitioner-see non-physician provider

Affordable Care Act-actually a shortened name for the Patient Protection and Affordable Care Act. See Patient Protection and Affordable Care Act.

American Academy of Emergency Physicians (AAEM)-AAEM is the specialty society of emergency medicine and the champion of the emergency physicians.[126]

> *"The Rape of Emergency Medicine* was first published anonymously by "The Phoenix" in 1992, as a quasi-fictional account of the physicians and patients harmed by egregious emergency medicine contract management group abuses. This engaging book was a catalyst for AAEM's formation, after the author, James Keaney, MD MPH FAAEM, revealed himself during a *60 Minutes* investigation of the abuses detailed in the book. Hundreds of emergency physicians, who had similar negative experiences and felt they were not properly represented by organized emergency medicine, contacted Dr. Keaney and began plans for what eventually became AAEM."[127]

American Board of Emergency Medicine (ABEM)- "The American Board of Emergency Medicine is one of 24 medical specialty certification boards recognized by the American Board of Medical Specialties. ABEM certifies emergency physicians who meet its educational, professional, and examination standards. ABEM certification is sought and earned by emergency physicians on a voluntary basis; ABEM is not a member association."[128] "It represents physicians' highest professional credential, reflecting that they have met an externally developed national standard."[129]

American College of Emergency Physicians (ACEP)-"The American College of Emergency Physicians is a professional organization of emergency medicine physicians in the United States."[130] Unlike the ABEM, the ACEP is not the certifying body that certifies emergency physicians as being board-certified. Membership in ACEP is optional and many board-certified emergency physicians elect to not become members. With few exceptions, one must pay an annual membership fee in to become a member and to maintain membership.

AMA-abbreviation for American Medical Association

American Medical Association (AMA)-the largest association of physicians in the United State. The AMA spends more of lobbying than any other medical society. Formed in the 1847, it has a membership of approximately 250,000. At one time (1950's) the AMA had approximately 75% of all practicing physicians as members. More recently, the percentage of practicing physicians who are members of the AMA is less than 25%.[131]

APP-abbreviation for Advanced Practice Practitioner

Benevolent Capitalism-a capitalistic system that uses its success to help people and/or society. In such a system, companies or their owners voluntarily use profits or the strength of their business for the good of people or society. Such "benevolence" is by choice, not forced upon them, and not done because of fear or risk of penalty. A person who practices benevolent capitalism is called a Benevolent Capitalist.

Co-Insurance- is a fee, typically stated as a percentage of a charge that the patient is responsible to pay. Assume a patient goes to a PCP and has a $25 co-pay and a 20% co-insurance. If the doctor is in-network and did a procedure that he bills $1000 in addition to his $150 office visit, the patient, or insured, would be required to pay a $25 co-pay to the PCP for the $150 PCP visit and then pay $200 more to the PCP for the patient's 20% portion of the $1,000 bill for the procedure, a total of $225.

Co-Pay-the amount the customer is required to pay in addition to the premiums and after the deductible has been paid in full. Co-pays are common. Often, the patient will have to pay the co-pay every time they see their PCP even if they have met their deductible. For example, a patient with a $25 co-pay on in-network primary care physician (PCP) visits and $50 on out of network PCPs goes to their PCP. If the PCP charges $150 for the visit, the patient will pay $25 and the insurer may be responsible for the remaining PCP visit charge.

Contract Management Group (CMG)-also known as a "staffing company," is typically a company that contracts with a hospital or other health care facility to provide a service to them i.e. professional services, and contracts with physicians or other non-physician providers, to provide the services on the CMG's behalf to the hospital or other health care facility. For example, a CMG contracts with a hospital to provide emergency staffing of the emergency department; the CMG recruits doctors to work in these ERs. The CMG gets paid a fee for this service in various forms i.e. cost plus a percentage, or a flat fee, or an hourly fee, or a fee determined by a formula that depends on number of hours, number of patients seen, various services provided, or a combination of these or other factors. Note when used in this book, the term CMG does not refer to the individual physicians or other NPP who provide services to patients who may work for CMGs. For the purposes of the discussions in this book, CMG refers to the ownership and management of the CMGs who may take advantage of their employees or workers by taking a significant portion of what the front line healthcare worker i.e. physician or NPP generates in revenue or establish or influence staffing models that may place physicians in an uncomfortable or dangerous situation or put patient care or safety at risk.

Deductible-the amount that the patient must pay before the insurance company will be responsible for any part of the healthcare costs by an insured customer. This is in addition to the policy premiums. Once a deductible is met, the patient often is still required to contribute a portion of the costs of their care i.e. co-pay, co-insurance, etc.

Diagnosis Diet (D-Diet)-meals that are created specific for people that have certain medical conditions. For example, there would be meals intended specifically for diabetics, kidney failure patients, heart patients, etc. The meals would be easily recognizable because of simple labeling. A color coded with a specific color for people with specific diagnoses, or a number range for a specific diagnosis or a combination of the two. For example, a diabetic would look for yellow labels and heart patients for a red label.

Diagnosis Meals (D-Meals)-See Diagnosis Diet

Direct Care Model-see Direct Care Organization

Direct Care Organization (DCO)-The Direct Care Organization (DCO) model is based on current payers of insurance (employers, employees and/or individuals) taking charge and arranging for or directly providing any healthcare that is needed by the members of the DCO i.e. employees, but can be owned or operated by anyone. The idea is to eliminate as many "middlemen" as possible that bring little to no value to the patients. The extreme DCO can provide every health service that is provided by any physician, hospital, or healthcare related facility. Others may offer less or offer a high deductible i.e. $100,000, catastrophic policy in the event the DCO could not provide a service or if costs of care would be excessive i.e. organ transplant, major trauma, etc. Would cover the physicians, specialists, imaging, labs, testing etc. as part of the membership and could have zero co-pays, deductibles etc. Any "profits" could go to the employer or employee as they are the "owners" of the DCO.

Drug Choice Act-A suggested regulation (not aware of any such law or act that currently exists) requiring big pharma, or anyone advertising pharmaceuticals, to not only disclose the prices of whatever they are advertising but also provide the names of 3 other drugs that can be used to treat the same condition or illness. To go further, the names of 3 of the most-commonly prescribed medications, along with the prices of each, and the names and prices of the 3 least expensive medications that can be used to treat the same condition or illness. Other suggested names for such a law are Drug Information Act or Drug Pricing Act.

Drug Information Act-See Drug Choice Act.

Drug Pricing Act-See Drug Choice Act.

Emergency Department (ED)-Area or department designated to take care of patients with medical emergencies. Ideally staffed with emergency physicians and other staff necessary to provide a high standard of care. Traditionally is a department within a hospital but more recently can be a separate entity/building i.e. Freestanding Emergency Centers. Often still referred to as "ER."

Emergency Medical Treatment and Labor Act (EMTALA)-In 1986, the emergency medical treatment and labor act known as EMTALA was passed. Essentially this law was meant to protect people when presenting to emergency departments, technically on hospital property or within so many feet of the hospital. It required any hospital that accepted governmental money i.e. Medicare, Medicaid or Tricare insurance to provide a medical screening exam to every patient who presents to the emergency department. The main thrust is that if someone has a medical emergency, the emergency department is required to treat the emergency within the capabilities of that facility regardless of the patient's ability to pay. To see the exact language, one can go to https://www.cms.gov/Regulations-and-Guidance/Legislation/EMTALA

Emergency Physician (EP)-a physician who has completed an emergency medicine residency and passed a formal board examination to become Board Certified by the American Board of Emergency Medicine (ABEM) or the American Board of Osteopathic Emergency Medicine (ABOEM). Any physician who works in an emergency department or ER is not necessarily an emergency physician unless they have the training and qualifications to be Board Certified by the American Board of Emergency Medicine or the American Board of Osteopathic Emergency Medicine.

Emergency Room (ER)-In the early days before emergency medicine became a recognized specialty, an emergency department (ED) may have been a single room. Hence the name, ER. While rarely are emergency departments a single room, the term ER is still sometimes used out of habit or because the term is more popular than the more proper term ED. Today most areas where emergency medicine is provided, the area where the public comes when they are having an emergency or acute unscheduled care and where emergency physicians work is called an emergency department (ED).

ER-abbreviation for emergency room-Still used by many as abbreviation for emergency department although technically not completely accurate reference.

Emergency Specialist-another term for an emergency physician

Employee Care Organization-similar to Employer Care Organization except has employee ownership. See Direct Care Organization.

Employer Care Organization (ECO)-Also referred to as an "ECO system" or employer care model (ECM). An ECO is one type of DCO. The employer owns and/or controls most of the healthcare that is provided to employee patients. This would include the medical practices i.e. PCPs, specialists, imaging equipment i.e. CT, MRI, ultrasound, etc., laboratory and testing equipment, etc. that are provided as part of "membership" or included for employees of the employer. ECOs can be owned by a single employer, a co-op or group of employers or even by employees.

Generic medication-copies of brand name drugs that have the same dosage, intended use, effects, side effects, route of administration, risks, safety, and strength as the original drug. In other words, their pharmacological effects are the same as those of their brand-name counterparts. May be differently shaped tablets or capsules, a different color or contain different preservatives than the original Brand Name medication. Often cost significantly less than the brand-named medications "equivalents"

Health Advisor-Someone who acts as an advisor, consultant, manager, or agent who understands, schedules, and handles just about everything related to health to help a person maximize health. Also called a Health Agent, Health Consultant, Health Manager.

Health Agent-See Health Advisor.

Health Consultant-See Health Advisor.

Health Manager-See Health Advisor.

Medical loss ratio (MLR)-Part of the Affordable Care Act (ACA) that requires a minimum percentage of every dollar paid in premiums to the insurer to be used by the insurance company on medical costs or quality improvement activities. The 80/20 rule requires at least 80 cents of every dollar paid in premium must be used to pay for medical costs or quality improvement activities.

Medical Menu-A listing of every procedure and service offered, including the retail price for each, along with the patient's insurance discounted price, the cash price if the patient has no insurance or chooses not to use their insurance, and the total amount that the patient will have to pay out-of-pocket that is in a clear, simple and easy to understand standardized manner.

Medication Menu-a list of every medication a pharmacy (or other dispenser of medications) sells to the public or uses in the care of patients, and the retail price should be available in print, like a restaurant menu. It should list medications in alphabetical order or by what diagnosis or condition that the medication is used to treat. The retail price should be listed and if a customer has insurance and enters their insurance information, it should list the price with that insurance including the total cost and the customer's portion or co-pay along with the pharmacy's, physician's or hospital's "cash" or "self-pay" price.

Midlevel Provider-term used for non-physician providers (NPP) that includes physician assistants (PA) and nurse practitioners (NPs). In the book NPP is used but could be substituted with midlevel. Some PAs and/or NPs do not like, or can even be insulted by, the term midlevel as they feel it does not appropriately represent them. Term is often still used by many in healthcare.

Mobile Medical Team (MMT)-specially trained health personnel, sent to the patient, in-person and onsite in patient's home or other location, with the backup of a physician specialist via telehealth. An example of this is DrHouseCallMD.com

Non-physician provider (NPP)-When used in this book, the term typically is referring to nurse practitioners (NPs) and physician assistants (PAs). The term APP, midlevel and or physician extender can also be used to represent NPs and PAs and has commonly been used in the past. In a broader or general sense, this term encompasses any or every person or entity that provides services that is not a physician. In addition to NPs and PAs, it would include other people that provide services such as psychologists, therapists, counselors etc. and non-humans such as hospitals, laboratories, imaging centers etc. that provide services to patients that are not physicians.

Nosocomial infections-These are infections that occur because one is in a hospital or other health care facility. It is an infection that a patient does not have before entering the hospital or health care facility.

NP-abbreviation for nurse practitioner

NPP-abbreviation for non-physician provider

Obamacare-a "nickname" or term commonly used to refer to the Patient Protection and Affordable Care Act.

PA-abbreviation for physician assistant

Patient Protection and Affordable Care Act-a.k.a. Affordable Care Act or ACA or Obamacare. Signed into law by then President Barrack Obama on March 23, 2010. Its intention was to lower the cost for low income households (100-400% of federal poverty level) to obtain healthcare by providing subsidies.

Point of Care (POC) testing-testing that occurs at or near the point of care without the need to send to an outside laboratory.

Policy Weakness Disclosure (PWD)-A disclosure that would require the insurer to point out the weaknesses of the policy the insurer is selling. Insurers would be required to clearly explain the policies and give the public disclosures of the both the good and bad aspects of the policy they are selling the public before they can sell it. This disclosure would be called a "Policy Weakness Disclosure".

Pre-Existing Condition-a condition that the insured has been treated for in the past or exists before the person is covered by the insurer.

Premium-the cost that is paid to have an insurance policy. This can be paid exclusively by the patient, the employer of the patient, someone else or any combination of the three. This is the minimum amount that the consumer will pay each year for healthcare. Most policies require the patient to pay additional money if care is needed i.e. deductible, co-pay, co-insurance, etc. Even if the insured does not require any treatment, medication or ever sees a doctor, the premium is paid.

Price-Quality Disclosure (P/Q Disclosure)-This is a name for a proposed disclosure that requires a hospital or other healthcare complex player to provide to the patient both the cost of services and the quality of the services the person(s) and entity providing services to the patient are, as measured by a standardized system. For example, a patient is admitted to the hospital to have gallbladder surgery. The total cost to the patient for all services from all parties involved for the surgery (price component). The Quality portion would require ratings of any physician or non-physician that may be involved in the patients care during that hospital stay including but not limited to the surgeon, the operating room staff (complication rate of both), radiologist(s) that may read imaging or tests, hospital quality standards such as hospital related infection rate (nosocomial) as compared to other hospitals, likelihood of falls, unexpected deaths, etc. The P/Q Disclosures are intended to force all in healthcare to be transparent and provide useful and valuable information to patients so they can make better-informed decisions.

Provider-a vague term referring to any person or entity (non-person) that provides services in healthcare. It includes but is not limited to physicians, PAs, NPs, hospitals, laboratories, imagining and diagnostic centers, therapists, or others who provide services within healthcare. It is recommended to avoid using this term as it can create confusion.

Staffing companies-Sometimes referred to as contract management groups (CMGs). See Contract Management Groups.

Vegan-Term used for someone who does not eat any animals or any products that come from animals. A vegan does not eat meat nor eggs, honey, milk, etc.

Vegetarian-Term used for someone who does not eat animals. Someone who does not eat meat of any kind. One can still eat products from animals i.e. milk, honey, etc. that does not cause the death of an animal and still be a vegetarian.

[1] Masterson, Les. June 23, 2019.
<https://www.healthcaredive.com/search/?q=health+insurance+premium+gro
wth+exceeds+wage+increases%2C+inflation >
[2] Masterson, Les. June 23, 2019.
<https://www.healthcaredive.com/search/?q=health+insurance+premium+gro
wth+exceeds+wage+increases%2C+inflation >
[3] Masterson, Les. June 23, 2019.
<https://www.healthcaredive.com/search/?q=health+insurance+premium+gro
wth+exceeds+wage+increases%2C+inflation >
[4] Masterson, Les. June 23, 2019.
<https://www.healthcaredive.com/search/?q=health+insurance+premium+gro
wth+exceeds+wage+increases%2C+inflation >
[5] *Centers for Medicare & Medicaid Services.* July 18, 2019. <
https://www.cms.gov/Research-Statistics-Data-and-Systems/Statistics-Trends-
and-
Reports/NationalHealthExpendData/Downloads/PieChartSourcesExpenditures.
pdf>
[6] *Committee for a Responsible Federal Budget.* July 18, 2019.
<https://www.crfb.org/papers/american-health-care-health-spending-and-
federal-budget>
[7] *Committee for a Responsible Federal Budget.* July 18, 2019.
<https://www.crfb.org/papers/american-health-care-health-spending-and-
federal-budget>
[8] United States Census Bureau. March 1, 2020. <
https://www.census.gov/popclock/>
[9] *Henry J. Kaiser Family Foundation.* March 1, 2020.
<http://files.kff.org/attachment/Report-Employer-Health-Benefits-Annual-
Survey-2018>
[10] Singh, Harshvardhan. June 19, 2019. <
https://medium.com/@harsh.singh.clif/u-s-health-care-ranked-worst-in-the-
developed-world-1d397cd291c6>
[11] *CNBC.* July 18, 2019. <https://www.cnbc.com/2018/03/22/the-real-reason-
medical-care-costs-so-much-more-in-the-us.html>
[12] *Henry J. Kaiser Family Foundation.* July 18, 2019.
[13] *Henry J. Kaiser Family Foundation.* July 18, 2019
[14] *Henry J. Kaiser Family Foundation.* July 18, 2019.
<http://files.kff.org/attachment/Report-Employer-Health-Benefits-Annual-
Survey-2018>
[15] *CNBC.* July 18, 2019. <https://www.cnbc.com/2018/01/31/health-insurer-
anthems-profit-2018-2018-forecast-top-estimates.html>

[16] Greene, Jay. July 18, 2019. <https://www.crainsdetroit.com/health-care/blue-cross-posts-2nd-highest-profit-past-decade>

[17] Mishra, Manas, Mathias, Tamara. July 18, 2019 <https://www.reuters.com/article/us-cigna-results/cigna-boosts-2018-forecast-after-third-quarter-earnings-beat-idUSKCN1N64GT>

[18] *Reuters*. July 18, 2019. < https://www.reuters.com/article/us-humana-results/humana-profit-tops-estimates-sees-550-million-tax-benefit-idUSKBN1FR1LR >

[19] Mishra, Manas, Mathias, Tamara. July 18, 2019 <https://www.reuters.com/article/us-cigna-results/cigna-boosts-2018-forecast-after-third-quarter-earnings-beat-idUSKCN1N64GT>

[20] Haefner, Morgan. June 20, 2019. <https://www.beckershospitalreview.com/payer-issues/america-s-largest-health-insurers-in-2018.html>

[21] Forbes List of top 20 Companies in Revenue. August 27, 2019. < https://fortune.com/fortune500/>

[22] *Salary.com* website. July 18, 2019. <https://www1.salary.com/UNITEDHEALTH-GROUP-INC-Executive-Salaries.html>

[23] Haefner, Morgan. July 18, 2019. <https://www.beckershospitalreview.com/payer-issues/unitedhealth-ceo-s-2018-compensation-21-5m.html>

[24] Sturdevant, Mathew. June 23, 2019. <http://www.courant.com/business/hc-united-health-group-ceo-pay-20150407-story.html>

[25] Mcgrath, Maggie. July 18, 2019. <https://www.forbes.com/sites/maggiemcgrath/2016/01/06/63-of-americans-dont-have-enough-savings-to-cover-a-500-emergency/#2c3ff4c34e0d>

[26] Bahney, Anna. July 18, 2019. <https://money.cnn.com/2018/05/22/pf/emergency-expenses-household-finances/index.html>

[27] Rosenbaum, Eric. July 18, 2019. <https://www.cnbc.com/2019/05/23/millions-of-americans-are-only-400-away-from-financial-hardship.html>

[28] Weyl, Ben. August 27, 2019. < https://www.commonwealthfund.org/publications/newsletter-article/americans-facing-increasing-problems-medical-debts>

[29] American College of Emergency Physicians. Leadership Advocacy Conference. May 5-8, 2019.

[30] Christensen-Garcia, Laura. August 12, 2019 < https://thefinancialclinic.org/medical-debt-collection-know-your-rights/>
[31] Weyl, Ben. August 27, 2019. < https://www.commonwealthfund.org/publications/newsletter-article/americans-facing-increasing-problems-medical-debts>
[32] Allen, Marshall. July 18, 2019. <https://www,npr.org/sections/health-shots/2018/05/25/613685732/why-your-health-insurer-doesnt-care-about-your-big-bills>
[33] Allen, Marshall. July 18, 2019. <https://www,npr.org/sections/health-shots/2018/05/25/613685732/why-your-health-insurer-doesnt-care-about-your-big-bills>
[34] Evers-Hillstrom, Karl. August 28, 2019. <https://www.opensecrets.org/news/2019/01/lobbying-spending-reaches-3-4-billion-in-18/>
[35] Policygenius.com June 19, 2019.
[36] Policygenius.com June 19, 2019.
[37] Policygenius.com, August 12, 2019. <https://www.policygenius.com/life-insurance/learn/whole-life-versus-term-life-insurance/>
[38] Ramsey, Dave. August 28, 2019. <https://www.youtube.com/watch?v=c4lnaZJKGvU>
[39] Ramsey, Dave. August 28, 2019. <https://www.youtube.com/watch?v=c4lnaZJKGvU>
[40] Royal PH.D., James, O'Shea, Arielle. April 10, 2020. <https://www.nerdwallet.com/blog/investing/average-stock-market-return/>
[41] *Henry J. Kaiser Family Foundation*. July 18, 2019. <http://files.kff.org/attachment/Report-Employer-Health-Benefits-Annual-Survey-2018>
[42] *Henry J. Kaiser Family Foundation*. July 18, 2019. <http://files.kff.org/attachment/Report-Employer-Health-Benefits-Annual-Survey-2018>
[43] *Henry J. Kaiser Family Foundation*. July 18, 2019. <http://files.kff.org/attachment/Report-Employer-Health-Benefits-Annual-Survey-2018>
[44] *Centers for Medicare & Medicaid Services*. July 18, 2019. < https://www.cms.gov/Research-Statistics-Data-and-Systems/Statistics-Trends-and-Reports/NationalHealthExpendData/Downloads/PieChartSourcesExpenditures.pdf>
[45] WebMD.com, February 9, 2020. < https://www.webmd.com/cancer/can-ct-scans-lead-to-cancer#1>
[46] WebMD.com, February 9, 2020. < https://www.webmd.com/cancer/can-ct-scans-lead-to-cancer#1>

[47] Indeed.com, June 26, 2019. <https://www.indeed.com/salaries/Primary-Care-Physician-Salaries>

[48] Meyers, Susan. December 8, 2019. <http://www.ed-qual.com/Emergency_Medicine_News/ED_News_ED_Outsourcing_Article.htm>

[49] AAEM.org, December 8, 2019. < https://www.aaem.org/about-us/our-values>

[50] ACEP.org, January 5, 2020. < https://www.acep.org/patient-care/policy-statements/definition-of-an-emergency-physician/>

[51] AAEM.org, December 7, 2019. < https://www.aaem.org/about-us/our-values>

[52] Daley, Robert & Post, Ted. (1973) *Magnum Force*. USA

[53] Sbeglia, Catherine. June 26, 2019. <https://www.rdmag.com/data-focus/2018/09/top-25-global-pharmaceutical-companies-market-cap-2018>

[54] Speights, Keith. July 18, 2019. <https://www.fool.com/investing/2016/07/31/12-big-pharma-stats-that-will-blow-you-away-aspx>

[55] Cox, Kate. June 25, 2019. < https://www.consumerreports.org/consumerist/what-are-the-10-biggest-money-making-prescription-drugs-and-what-do-they-treat/>

[56] Drugbank. August 30, 2019. < https://www.drugbank.ca/stats>

[57] Johnson, Linda A. June 25, 2019. <https://medicalxpress.com/news/2019-05-fda-2m-medicine-expensive.html>

[58] Terry, Mark. March 10, 2020. < https://www.biospace.com/article/drug-pricing-watchdog-thinks-biogen-s-spinraza-should-be-cheaper/>

[59] Crawford, Chris. January 27, 2020. <https://www.aafp.org/news/health-of-the-public/20140428nonadherencestudy.html>

[60] Brody, Jane E. January 27, 2020. <https://www.nytimes.com/2017/04/17/well/the-cost-of-not-taking-your-medicine.html>

[61] Rowan, Karen. January 27, 2020. <https://www.livescience.com/23179-why-americans-prescriptions-are-going-unfilled.html>

[62] Miller, Emily. June 25, 2019. <https://www.drugwatch.com/featured/us-drug-prices-higher-vs-world/>

[63] Brody, Jane E. April 24, 2020. <https://www.nytimes.com/2017/04/17/well/the-cost-of-not-taking-your-medicine.html >

[64] Speights, Keith. July 18, 2019. <https://www.fool.com/investing/2016/07/31/12-big-pharma-stas-that-will-blow-you-away-aspx>

[65] Speights, Keith. July 18, 2019. <https://www.fool.com/investing/2016/07/31/12-big-pharma-stas-that-will-blow-you-away-aspx>

[66] Miller, Emily. June 25, 2019. <https://www.drugwatch.com/featured/us-drug-prices-higher-vs-world/>

[67] Miller, Emily. June 25, 2019. <https://www.drugwatch.com/featured/us-drug-prices-higher-vs-world/>

[68] Miller, Emily. June 25, 2019. <https://www.drugwatch.com/featured/us-drug-prices-higher-vs-world/>

[69] Johnson, Linda A.. June 25, 2019. <https://medicalxpress.com/news/2019-05-fda-2m-medicine-expensive.html

[70] Miller, Emily. June 25, 2019. <https://www.drugwatch.com/featured/us-drug-prices-higher-vs-world/>

[71] Johnson, Linda A.. June 25, 2019. <https://medicalxpress.com/news/2019-05-fda-2m-medicine-expensive.html

[72] Speights, Keith. July 18, 2019. <https://www.fool.com/investing/2016/07/31/12-big-pharma-stas-that-will-blow-you-away-aspx>

[73] WebMD. March 16, 2020. < https://www.webmd.com/healthy-aging/generic-drugs-answers-to-common-questions#1>

[74] Stoppler, M.D., Melissa. July 15, 2019. <https://www.medicinenet.com/generic_drugs_are_they_as_good_as_brand-names/views.htm>

[75] GoodRX.com. July 7, 2019. < https://www.goodrx.com/>

[76] Zwillich, Todd. March 10, 2020. <https://www.webmd.com/arthritis/news/20050407/bextra-taken-off-market-celebrex-gets-warning#1>

[77] Jaffe, Susan. July 18, 2019. <https://khn.org/news/no-more-secrets-congress-bans-pharmacist-gag-orders-on-drug-prices/>

[78] Jaffe, Susan. July 18, 2019. <https://khn.org/news/no-more-secrets-congress-bans-pharmacist-gag-orders-on-drug-prices/>

[79] Jaffe, Susan. July 18, 2019. <https://khn.org/news/no-more-secrets-congress-bans-pharmacist-gag-orders-on-drug-prices/>

[80] *Committee for a Responsible Federal Budget.* July 18, 2019. <https://www.crfb.org/papers/american-health-care-health-spending-and-federal-budget>

[81] Haefner, Morgan. June 20, 2019. <https://www.beckershospitalreview.com/payer-issues/america-s-largest-health-insurers-in-2018.html>

[82] Miller, Emily. July 18, 2019. <https://www.drugwatch.com/featured/us-drug-prices-higher-vs-world/>

[83] Li, Victor. August 29, 2019. < http://www.abajournal.com/magazine/article/legal_advertising_viral_video>

[84] U.S. Chamber, Institute for Legal Reform. August 29, 2019. <https://www.instituteforlegalreform.com/research/trial-lawyer-ad>

[85] Torrey, Trisha. August 29, 2019. <
https://www.verywellhealth.com/defensive-medicine-2615160>
[86] Vinocur M.D., Leigh. July 18, 2019.
<https://www.huffpost.com/entry/trauma-care-will-it-be-there_b_809069>
[87] Gorman, Tom. July 18, 2019. <https://latimes.com/archives/la-xpm-2002-jul-03-na-trauma3-story.html>
[88] Vinocur M.D., Leigh. July 18, 2019.
<https://www.huffpost.com/entry/trauma-care-will-it-be-there_b_809069>
[89] *Centers for Medicare & Medicaid Services.* July 18, 2019.
<https://www.cms.gov/Outreach-and-Education/Medicare-Learning-Network-MLN/MLNProducts/Downloads/Telehealth-Services-Text-Only.pdf>
[90] Haberkorn, Jennifer. August 12, 2019.
<https://www.healthaffairs.org/do/10.1377/hpb20101112.449011/full/>
[91] *Center for Disease Control.* July 18, 2019.
<https://www.cdc.gov/tobacco/data_statistics/fact_sheet/economics/econ_facts/index.htm>
[92] *Center for Disease Control.* July 18, 2019.
<https://www.cdc.gov/tobacco/data_statistics/fact_sheet/economics/econ_facts/index.htm>
[93] *Henry J. Kaiser Family Foundation.* July 18, 2019.
<http://files.kff.org/attachment/Report-Employer-Health-Benefits-Annual-Survey-2018>
[94] *United Poultry Concerns.* July 1, 2019. <https://www.upc-online.org/slaughter/2008americans.html>
[95] *Animal Matters.* July 1, 2019. <http://www.animalmatters.org/facts/farm/>
[96] Charlton, Corey. December 11, 2019. <
https://www.dailymail.co.uk/news/article-3211443/All-ground-beef-eaten-U-S-contains-fecal-contamination-Study-reveals-dangers-poisoning-meat-not-properly-cooked.html>
[97] *Skeptical Science.* August 13, 2019. <https://skepticalscience.com/how-much-meat-contribute-to-gw.html>
[98] Forks over Knives Documentary, Director Lee Fulkerson, Netflix 2011.
[99] *What the Health* Documentary, Directors Kip Anderson and Keegan Kuhn, Netflix 2017.
[100] *What the Health* Documentary, Directors Kip Anderson and Keegan Kuhn, Netflix 2017.
[101] *Forks over Knives* Documentary, Director Lee Fulkerson, Netflix 2011.
[102] *Forks over Knives* Documentary, Director Lee Fulkerson, Netflix 2011.
[103] Tomaselli, Paige. *What the Health* Documentary, Directors Kip Anderson and Keegan Kuhn, Netflix 2017

[104] Tomaselli, Paige. *What the Health* Documentary, Directors Kip Anderson and Keegan Kuhn, Netflix 2017.

[105] Statista. March 14, 2020. < https://www.statista.com/statistics/502286/global-meat-and-seafood-market-value/>

[106] *What the Health* Documentary, Directors Kip Anderson and Keegan Kuhn, Netflix 2017>

[107] Sass MPH, RD, Cynthia. July 18, 2019. <https://www.health.com/nutrition/yes-the-bacon-cancer-link-is-real-but-heres-why-you-shouldnt-freak-out>

[108] *World Health Organization*. July 4, 2019. <https://www.who.int/features/qa/cancer-red-meat/en/>

[109] *What the Health* Documentary, Directors Kip Anderson and Keegan Kuhn, Netflix 2017.

[110] *World Health Organization*. July 4, 2019. <https://www.who.int/features/qa/cancer-red-meat/en/>

[111] Esselstyn, M.D., Caldwell. *Forks over Knives* Documentary, Director Lee Fulkerson, Netflix 2011.

[112] Greger, M.D., Michael. *What the Health* Documentary, Directors Kip Anderson and Keegan Kuhn, Netflix 2017.

[113] *Interaction Design Foundation*. August 13, 2019. <https://www.interaction-design.org/literature/article/kiss-keep-it-simple-stupid-a-design-principle>

[114] *Centers for Medicare & Medicaid Services*. July 4, 2019. <https://innovation.cms.gov/initiatives/et3/>

[115] Center for Disease Control and Prevention. March 15, 2020. < https://www.cdc.gov/coronavirus/2019-ncov/cases-in-us.html>

[116] Alonso-Zaldivar, Ricardo. March 15, 2020. <https://abcnews.go.com/Health/wireStory/coronavirus-spreads-medicare-telemedicine-option-69441233>

[117] Office of the Texas Governor. March 16, 2020. < https://gov.texas.gov/news/post/governor-abbott-tdi-ask-health-insurance-providers-to-waive-costs-associated-with-coronavirus>

[118] New York State Governor. March 15, 2020. < https://www.governor.ny.gov/news/during-coronavirus-briefing-governor-cuomo-announces-department-financial-services-will-require>

[119] Hale, Conor. December 11, 2019. < https://www.fiercebiotech.com/medtech/google-s-cancer-spotting-ai-outperforms-radiologists-reading-lung-ct-scans>

[120] Massingale, Lynn. ACEP Legislative & Advocacy Conference. Washington DC. May 2019.

[121] Suderman, Peter. Retrieved August 31, 2019. < https://reason.com/2019/07/17/bernie-sanders-medicare-for-all-cost-40-trillion-obamacare-single-payer/>

[122] Committee for a Responsible Federal Budget. Retrieved August 31, 2019. <
https://www.crfb.org/blogs/how-much-will-medicare-all-cost>
[123] Suderman, Peter. Retrieved August 31, 2019. <
https://reason.com/2019/07/17/bernie-sanders-medicare-for-all-cost-40-
trillion-obamacare-single-payer/>
[124] Kaiser Health News. Retrieved August 31, 2019. <
https://khn.org/news/delaneys-debate-claim-that-medicare-for-all-will-
shutter-hospitals-goes-overboard/>
[125] Ellison, Ayla. Retrieved August 31, 2019.
<https://www.beckershospitalreview.com/finance/medicare-for-all-would-
force-colorado-hospital-to-close-cfo-says.html?origin=cfoe&utm_source=cfoe>
[126] American Academy of Emergency Medicine. March 23, 2020. <
https://www.aaem.org/>
[127] AAEM website. May 1, 2020. < https://www.aaem.org/about-us/our-
values/history>
[128] Bing.com. March 23, 2020. <
https://www.bing.com/search?q=abem&form=EDGEAR&qs=PF&cvid=1bd8c53
d67904b32a52cee33f8338ec5&cc=US&setlang=en-US&plvar=0&PC=HCTS>
[129] American Board of Emergency Medicine. March 23, 2020. <
https://www.abem.org/public/>
[130] Bing.com. March 23, 2020.
<https://www.bing.com/search?q=acep&qs=n&form=QBRE&sp=-
1&ghc=1&pq=acep&sc=8-
4&sk=&cvid=132A5316875C4AB09FB9E2D36F909A71>
[125] Graham, Judith. May 1, 2020. <https://www.businessinsider.com/doctors-
american-medical-association-2016-12>

REFERENCES

Masterson, Les. (2018, October 4). *Health insurance premium growth exceeds wage increases, inflation.* Retrieved June 23, 2019, from https://www.healthcaredive.com/search/?q=health+insurance+premium+grow th+exceeds+wage+increases%2C+ inflation

Committee for a Responsible Federal Budget. (2018, May 16). *American Health Care: Health Spending and the Federal Budget.* Retrieved July 18, 2019, from https://www.crfb.org/papers/american-health-care-health-spending-and-federal-budget

Centers for Medicare & Medicaid Services, Office of the Actuary, National Health Statistics Group. (No date). *The Nation's Health Dollar ($3.5 Trillion), Calendar Year 2017, Where it Went.* Retrieved July 18, 2019, from https://www.cms.gov/Research-Statistics-Data-and-Systems/Statistics-Trends-and-Reports/ NationalHealthExpendData/Downloads/PieChartSourcesExpenditures.pdf

Singh, Harshvardhan. (2018, April 13). *U.S. Health Care Ranked Worst in the Developed World.* Retrieved June 19, 2019, from https://medium.com/@harsh.singh.clif/u-s-health-care-ranked-worst-in-the-developed-world-1d397cd291c6

CNBC. (2018, March 22, updated 2018, September 3). *Here's the real reason health care costs so much more in the US.* Retrieved July 18, 2019, from https://www.cnbc.com/2018/03/22/the-real-reason-medical-care-costs-so-much-more-in-the-us.html

The Henry J. Kaiser Family Foundation. (2018). *Employer Health Benefits, 2018 Summary of Findings.* Retrieved July 18, 2019, from http://files.kff.org/attachment/Report-Employer-Health-Benefits-Annual-Survey-2018

Coombs, Bertha. (2017, August 5, updated 2017, August 6). *As Obamacare twists in political winds, top insurers made $6 billion (not that there is anything wrong with that).* Retrieved July 18, 2019, from https://www.cnbc.com/2017/08/05/top-health-insurers-profit-surge-29-percent-to-6-billion-dollars.html
Reuters published on CNBC website. (2018, January 31). *Health insurer Anthem's profit, 2018 forecast top estimates.* Retrieved July 18, 2019, from https://www.cnbc.com/2018/01/31/health-insurer-anthems-profit-2018-2018-forecast-top-estimates.html

Greene, Jay. (2019, March 1). *Blue Cross posts 2nd-highest profit in past decade.* Retrieved July 18, 2019, from https://www.crainsdetroit.com/health-care/blue-cross-posts-2nd-highest-profit-past-decade

Mishra, Manas et al. (2018, November 1). *Cigna boosts 2018 forecast after third quarter earnings beat.* Retrieved July 18, 2019, from https://www.reuters.com/article/us-cigna-results/cigna-boosts-2018-forecast-after-third-quarter-earnings-beat-idUSKCN1N64GT

Reuters. (2018, February 7). *Humana profits tops estimates; see $550 million tax benefit.* Retrieved July 18, 2019, from https://www.reuters.com/article/us-humana-results/humana-profit-tops-estimates-sees-550-million-tax-benefit-idUSKBN1FR1LR

Google. (2018, November 8). *Search of: What percentage of healthcare premiums do employers pay?* Retrieved August 21, 2019, from https://www.google.com/search?source=hp&ei=72FdXdiINsnQsAXVjKfwDw&q=what+percentage+of+premiums+do+employers+pay&oq=what+percentage+of+premiums+do+employers+pay&gs_l=psy-ab.3..0j0i22i30l2.2772.14635..15205...1.0..0.588.6625.14j25j3j3j0j1....2..0....1..gws-wiz.......0i70i251j0i10.ROQMWzhcioc&ved=0ahUKEwiYvJq9opTkAhVJKKwKHVXGCf4Q4dUDCAc&uact=5

Google. (No date). *Search of: What percentage of insurance premiums are paid out in claims?* Retrieved August 21, 2019, from https://www.google.com/search?ei=AWJdXf7bDtC8sAWloL6YDg&q=what+percentage+of+insurance+premiums+are+paid+out+in+claims%3F&oq=what+percentage+of+insurance+premiums+are+paid+out+in+claims%3F&gs_l=psy-ab.3..0i22i30.255279.272832..273295...1.2..0.267.5045.19j23j2......0....1..gws-wiz.......0i71j0i13j0i8i7i30j0i8i30j0.WxrUKqWLapc&ved=0ahUKEwi-4L3FopTkAhVQHqwKHSWQD-MQ4dUDCAo&uact=5

Haefner, Morgan. (2019, January 10). *America's largest health insurers in 2018.* Retrieved June 20, 2019, from https://www.beckershospitalreview.com/payer-issues/america-s-largest-health-insurers-in-2018.html

Salary.com. (no date). *UNITEDHEALTH GROUP INC, Compensation by Company.* Retrieved July 18, 2019, from https://www1.salary.com/UNITEDHEALTH-GROUP-INC-Executive-Salaries.html

Haefner, Morgan. (2019, April 23). *UnitedHealth CEO's 2018 compensation: $21,5M.* Retrieved July 18, 2019, from https://www.beckershospitalreview.com/payer-issues/unitedhealth-ceo-s-2018-compensation-21-5m.html

McGrath, Maggie. (No date). *63% Of Americans Don't Have Enough Savings To Cover A $500 Emergency.* Retrieved July 18, 2019, from https://www.forbes.com/sites/maggiemcgrath/2016/01/06/63-of-americans-dont-have-enough-savings-to-cover-a-500-emergency/#2c3ff4c34e0d

Bahney, Anna. (2018, May 22). *40% of Americans can't cover a $400 emergency expense.* Retrieved July 18, 2019, from https://money.cnn.com/2018/05/22/pf/emergency-expenses-household-finances/index.html

Rosenbaum, Eric. (2019, May 23). *Millions of Americans are only $400 away from financial hardship. Here's why.* Retrieved July 18, 2019, from https://www.cnbc.com/2019/05/23/millions-of-americans-are-only-400-away-from-financial-hardship.html

Pollitz, Karen et al. (2019, June 20). *An Examination of Surprise Medical Bills and Proposals to Protect Consumers from Them.* Retrieved August 21, 2019 from https://www.kff.org/health-costs/issue-brief/an-examination-of-surprise-medical-bills-and-proposals-to-protect-consumers-from-them/
Allen, Marshall. (2018, May 25). *Why Your Health Insurer Doesn't Care About Your Big Bills.* Retrieved July 18, 2019, from https://www,npr.org/sections/health-shots/2018/05/25/613685732/why-your-health-insurer-doesnt-care-about-your-big-bills

Fortune Media IP Limited. (No date). *THE TOP 10.* Retrieved August 21, 2019, from https://fortune.com/fortune500/

Miller, Emily. (2018, January 25). *US Drug Prices vs The World.* Retrieved June 25, 2019, from https://www.drugwatch.com/featured/us-drug-prices-higher-vs-world/

Jaffe, Susan. (2018, October 10). *No More Secrets: Congress Bans Pharmacist "Gag Orders" On Drug Prices.* Retrieved https://khn.org/news/no-more-secrets-congress-bans-pharmacist-gag-orders-on-drug-prices/

Vinocur, M.D., Leigh. (2011, January 19, updated 2011, May 25). *Trauma Care: Will It Be There When You Need It?* Retrieved July 18, 2019, from https://www.huffpost.com/entry/trauma-care-will-it-be-there_b_809069

Gorman, Tom. (2002, July 3). *Vegas' Only Trauma Unit to Close Today.* Retrieved July 18, 2019, from https://latimes.com/archives/la-xpm-2002-jul-03-na-trauma3-story.html

Centers for Medicare & Medicaid Services. (No date). *Medicare Learning Network: Telehealth Services.* Retrieved July 18, 2019 from https://www.cms.gov/Outreach-and-Education/Medicare-Learning-Network-MLN/MLNProducts/Downloads/Telehealth-Services-Text-Only.pdf

Haberkorn, Jennifer. (2010, November 12). *Medial Loss Ratios. Health insurers will soon be required to spend a specific share of the premiums they collect on health care for policyholders.* Retrieved August 21, 2019, from https://www.healthaffairs.org/do/10.1377/hpb20101112.449011/full

Sbeglia, Catherine. (2018, September 17). *Top 25 Global Pharmaceutical Companies by Market Cap 2018.* Retrieved June 26, 2019, from https://www.rdmag.com/data-focus/2018/09/top-25-global-pharmaceutical-companies-market-cap-2018

Speights, Keith. (2016, July 31). *12 Big Pharma Stata That Will Blow You Away. Big Pharma means big numbers—usually. But there are some small numbers that are fascinating, too.* Retrieved July 18, 2019, from https://www.fool.com/investing/2016/07/31/12-big-pharma-stats-that-will-blow-you-away-aspx

Cox, Kate. (2017, September 26). *What Are The 10 Biggest Money-Making Prescription Drugs, And What Do They Treat?* Retrieved June 25, 2019, from https://www.consumerreports.org/consumerist/what-are-the-10-biggest-money-making-prescription-drugs-and-what-do-they-treat/

Johnson, Linda A. (2019, May 24). *FDA approves $2M medicine, most expensive ever.* Retrieved June 25, 2019, from https://medicalxpress.com/news/2019-05-fda-2m-medicine-expensive.html

The Business Research Company. (2018, May 16). *The Growing Pharmaceuticals Market: Expert Forecasts and Analysis.* Retrieved July, 18, 2019, from https://blog.marketresearch.com/the-growing-pharmaceuticals-market-expert-forecasts-and-analysis

Jena, Dr. Anupam B. (2018, January 19). *US drug prices higher than in the rest of the world, here's why.* Retrieved July 18, 2019, from https://thehill.com/opinion/healthcare/369727-us-drug-prices-higher-than-in-the-rest-of-the-world-heres-why

Center for Disease Control and Prevention. (No date). *Economic Trends in Tobacco.* (No date). Retrieved July 18, 2019, from https://www.cdc.gov/tobacco/data_statistics/fact_sheets/economics/econ_fac ts/index.htm

United Poultry Concerns. (2009, October 22). *Average and Total Number of Animals Who Died to Feed Americans in 2008.* Retrieved July 1, 2019, from https://www.upc-online.org/slaughter/2008americans.html

Animal Matters. (No date). *Facts-Farm Animals.* Retrieved July 1, 2019, from http://www.animalmatters.org/facts/farm

Sass, MPH, RD, Cynthia. (2018, March 30). *Yes, the Bacon-Cancer Link Is Real, But Here's Why You Shouldn't Freak Out.* Retrieved July 18, 2019, from https://www.health.com/nutrition/yes-the-bacon-cancer-link-is-real-but-heres-why-you-shouldnt-freak-out

World Health Organization. (2015, October). *Q&A on the carcinogenicity of the consumption of red meat and processed meat.* Retrieved July 4, 2019, from https://www.who.int/features/qa/cancer-red-meat/en/

International Insurance.com. (No date). *Ranking the Top Healthcare Systems by Country.* Retrieved June 19, 2019, from https://www.internationalinsurance.com/health/systems/

National Conference of State Legislatures. (2018, December 4). *Health Insurance: Premiums and Increases.* Retrieved June 19, 2019, from http://www.ncsl.org/research/health/health-insurance-premiums.aspx

Ellis, Monique. (2019, March 20). *Who are the top 10 pharmaceutical companies in the world? (2019).* Retrieved August 21, 2019, from https://www.proclinical.com/blogs/2019-3/the-top-10-pharmaceutical-companies-in-the-world-2019

Christensen-Garcia, Laura. (2018, April 30). *Medical Debt Collection: Know Your Rights.* Retrieved August 21, 2019, from https://thefinancialclinic.org/medical-debt-collection-know-your-rights/

Indeed.com. (2019, June 17). *Primary Care Physician Salaries in the United States.* Retrieved June 26, 2019, from https://www.indeed.com/salaries/Primary-Care-Physician-Salaries

Weber, David Ollier. (2019, February 11). *How Many Patients Can a Primary Care Physician Treat?* Retrieved June 26, 2019, from https://www.physicianleaders.org/news/how-many-patients-can-primary-care-physician-treat

Berlin, Joey. (2018, September). *Coming of Age: Celebrating 15 Years of Texas Tort Reform.* Retrieved August 21, 2019, from https://www.texmed.org/Template.aspx?id=48427

Fiorillo, Steve. (2019, February 3). *What is the Average Income in the U.S. in 2019?* Retrieved July 4, 2019, from https://www.thestreet.com/personal-finance/average-income-in-us-14852178

Centers for Medicare & Medicaid Services. (No date). *Emergency Triage, Treat, and Transport (ET3) Model.* Retrieved July 4, 2019, from https://innovation.cms.gov/initiatives/et3/

Stoppler, M.D., Melissa. (No date). *Generic Drugs, Are They as Good as Brand Names?* Retrieved July 15, 2019, from https://www.medicinenet.com/generic_drugs_are_they_as_good_as_brand-names/views.htm
Sturdevant, Matthew. (2015, April 7). *UnitedHealth Group CEO's Compensation Was $66.13 Million Last Year.* Retrieved June 23, 2019, from http://www.courant.com/business/hc-united-health-group-ceo-pay-20150407-story.html

Policygenius.com. Retrieved June 19, 2019.

Centers for Medicare & Medicaid Services, The Center for Consumer Information & Insurance Oversight. (No date). *Medical Loss Ratio: Getting Your Money's Worth on Health Insurance.* Retrieved June 23, 2019, from https://www.cms.gov/CCIIO/Resources/Fact-Sheets-and-FAQs/mlrfinalrule.html

Hankin, Aaron. (2018, October 29). *How U.S. Healthcare Costs Compare to Other Countries.* Retrieved August 21, 2019, from https://www.investopedia.com/articles/personal-finance/072116/us-healthcare-costs-compared-other-countries.asp

Ratini, DO, MS, Melinda. (2019, February 1). *What You Should Know About Processed Meat.* Retrieved July 15, 2019, from https://www.webmd.com/food-recipes/ss/slideshow-processed-meats

Reinagel, Monica. (2016, August 2). *What's the Definition of Processed Meat?* Retrieved July 15, 2019, from https://www.scientificamerican.com/article/what-s-the-definition-of-processed-meat/

Fry, MS, RD, Sidney. (2015, June 3, updated 2018, April 6). *What Is a "Processed" Food?* Retrieved July 15, 2019, from https://www.cookinglight.com/eating-smart/smart-choices/what-are-processed-foods

BBC. (2015, October 26). *What is processed meat?* Retrieved July 15, 2019, from https://www.bbc.com/news/health-34620617

Marsh, Tori. (2019, March 8). *The 20 Most Expensive Outpatient Drugs in the U.S.A.* Retrieved August 22, 2019, from https://www.goodrx.com/blog/20-most-expensive-drugs-in-the-usa/

Healthcare.gov. (no date). *Health insurance rights & protections Rate Review & the 80/20 Rule.* Retrieved June 23, 2019, from https://www.healthcare.gov/health-care-law-protections/rate-review/

Berger, Rob. (2018, July 4). *Shouldn't Life Insurance Companies All Be Bankrupt?* Retrieved August 22, 2019, from https://www.doughroller.net/insurance/life-insurance/shouldnt-life-insurance-companies-all-be-bankrupt/

Berchick, Edward R. et al. (2018, September 12). *Health Insurance Coverage in the United States: 2017.* Retrieved June 19, 2019, from https://www.census.gov/content/dam/Census/library/publications/2018/demo/p60-264.pdf

Sherman, Erik. (2019, February 21). *U.S. Health Care Costs Skyrocketed to $3.65 Trillion in 2018.* Retrieved August 22, 2019, from https://fortune.com/2019/02/21/us-health-care-costs-2/

Gould, Elise. (2012, December 5). *EMPLOYER-SPONSORED HEALTH INSURANCE COVERAGE CONTINUES TO DECLINE IN A NEW DECADE.* Economic Policy Institute. Retrieved August 22, 2019, from https://www.epi.org/publication/bp353-employer-sponsored-health-insurance-coverage/

The Commonwealth Fund. (No date). *Survey: 79 Million Americans Have Problems with Medical Bills or Debt.* Retrieved June 26, 2019, from https://www.commonwealthfund.org/publications/newsletter-article/survey-79-million-americans-have-problems-medical-bills-or-debt

Horton, Melissa. (2018, September 25). *Average Cost of Health Insurance.* Retrieved August 22, 2019, from https://lendedu.com/blog/average-cost-of-health-insurance/

Reid, T.R. (2017, June 17). *How We Spend $3,400,000,000,000. Why more than half of America's healthcare spending goes to five percent of patients.* Retrieved June 19, 2019, from https://www.theatlantic.com/health/archive/2017/06/how-we-spend-3400000000000/530355/

Koba, Mark. (2011, September 12, updated 2011, September 13). *Why US Pays More for Health Care Than Other Nations.* Retrieved August 22, 2019, from https://www.cnbc.com/id/44180042

Gooch, Kelly. (2019, June 24). *Trump demands transparency on healthcare costs: 7 things to know.* Retrieved August 22, 2019, from https://www.beckershospitalreview.com/finance/trump-demands-transparency-on-healthcare-costs-7-things-to-know.html

Grand View Research, Inc. (2018, May 28). *Meat, Poultry & Seafood Market Size Worth $7.3 Trillion By 2025: Grand View Research, Inc.* Retrieved July 4, 2019, from https://www.prnewswire.com/news-releases/meat-poultry--seafood-market-size-worth-73-trillion-by-2025-grand-view-research-inc-683844731.html

Shahbandeh, M. (2019, January 17). *Global Meat Industry-Statistics & Facts.* Retrieved July 4, 2019, from https://www.statista.com/topics/4880/global-meat-industry/

American College of Emergency Physicians. Leadership & Advocacy Conference, Washington DC May 5-8, 2019.

Weyl, Ben. (2008, September 8). *Americans Facing Increasing Problems with Medical Debts.* Retrieved August 27, 2019, from https://www.commonwealthfund.org/publications/newsletter-article/americans-facing-increasing-problems-medical-debts

www.ingramcontent.com/pod-product-compliance
Lightning Source LLC
Chambersburg PA
CBHW020602270326
41927CB00005B/139